PROBLEM-BASED OBSTETRIC ULTRASOUND
ULTRASOUND

Second Edition

Series in Maternal-Fetal Medicine

About the Series

Published in association with the *Journal of Maternal Fetal and Neonatal Medicine*, the series in *Maternal Fetal Medicine* keeps readers up to date with the latest clinical therapies to improve the health of pregnant patients and ensure a successful birth. Each volume in the series is prepared separately and typically focuses on a topical theme. Volumes are published on an occasional basis, depending on the emergence of new developments.

Cesarean Delivery: A Comprehensive Illustrated Practical Guide
Gian Carlo Di Renzo, Antonio Malvasi

Obstetric Evidence Based Guidelines, Third Edition
Vincenzo Berghella

Maternal-Fetal Evidence Based Guidelines, Third Edition
Vincenzo Berghella

Maternal-Fetal and Obstetric Evidence Based Guidelines, Two Volume Set, Third Edition
Vincenzo Berghella

The Long-Term Impact of Medical Complications in Pregnancy: A Window into Maternal and Fetal Future Health
Eyal Sheiner

Operative Obstetrics, Fourth Edition
Joseph J. Apuzzio, Anthony M. Vintzileos, Vincenzo Berghella, Jesus R. Alvarez-Perez

Placenta Accreta Syndrome
Robert M. Silver

Neurology and Pregnancy: Clinical Management
Michael S. Marsh, Lina Nashef, Peter Brex

Fetal Cardiology: Embryology, Genetics, Physiology, Echocardiographic Evaluation, Diagnosis, and Perinatal Management of Cardiac Diseases, Third Edition
Simcha Yagel, Norman H. Silverman, Ulrich Gembruch

New Technologies and Perinatal Medicine: Prediction and Prevention of Pregnancy Complications
Moshe Hod, Vincenzo Berghella, Mary D'Alton, Gian Carlo Di Renzo, Eduard Gratacos, Vassilios Fanos

Problem-Based Obstetric Ultrasound, Second Edition
Amar Bhide, Asma Khalil, Aris T Papageorghiou, Susana Pereira, Shanthi Sairam, Basky Thilaganathan

For more information about this series please visit: https://www.crcpress.com/Series-in-Maternal-Fetal-Medicine/book-series/CRCSERMATFET

PROBLEM-BASED OBSTETRIC ULTRASOUND

Second Edition

Amar Bhide MD MRCOG
Consultant in Maternal-Fetal Medicine
Fetal Medicine Unit, St George's Hospital Medical School
London, UK

Asma Khalil MBBCh MD MRCOG MSc(Epi) DFSRH Dip(GUM)
Professor and Consultant in Fetal Medicine and Obstetrics
St George's University Hospitals
London, UK

Aris T Papageorghiou MRCOG
Consultant in Maternal-Fetal Medicine
Fetal Medicine Unit, St George's Hospital Medical School
London, UK

Susana Pereira MD
Consultant Obstetrician and Sub-specialist in Fetal Medicine
Kingston Hospital
London, UK

Shanthi Sairam MD MRCOG
Consultant OBGyn and Specialist in Fetal Medicine
Mediclinic City Hospital
Dubai, UAE

Basky Thilaganathan MD MRCOG
Professor and Director
Fetal Medicine Unit, St George's University Hospitals NHS Foundation Trust
London, UK

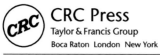

CRC Press
Taylor & Francis Group
Boca Raton London New York

CRC Press is an imprint of the
Taylor & Francis Group, an **informa** business

CRC Press
Taylor & Francis Group
6000 Broken Sound Parkway NW, Suite 300
Boca Raton, FL 33487-2742

© 2020 by Taylor & Francis Group, LLC
CRC Press is an imprint of Taylor & Francis Group, an Informa business

No claim to original U.S. Government works

Printed on acid-free paper

International Standard Book Number-13: 978-1-4987-0189-1 (Paperback)
978-0-367-40800-8 (Hardback)

Library of Congress Cataloging-in-Publication Data

Names: Bhide, Amarnath G., author.
Title: Problem-based obstetric ultrasound / Amar Bhide, Asma Khalil, Aris T. Papageorghiou, Susana Pereira, Shanthi Sairam, Basky Thilaganathan.
Other titles: Series in maternal-fetal medicine. 2158-0855
Description: Second edition. | Boca Raton : CRC Press, [2020] | Series: Series in maternal-fetal medicine | Preceded by Problem-based obstetric ultrasound / Basky Thilaganathan ... [et al.]. 2007. | Includes bibliographical references and index.
Identifiers: LCCN 2019034447 (print) | LCCN 2019034448 (ebook) | ISBN 9781498701891 (paperback ; alk. paper) | ISBN 9780367408008 (hardback ; alk. paper) | ISBN 9780429156694 (ebook)
Subjects: MESH: Ultrasonography, Prenatal--methods | Pregnancy Complications--diagnostic imaging
Classification: LCC RG527.5.U48 (print) | LCC RG527.5.U48 (ebook) | NLM WQ 209 | DDC 618.2/07543--dc23
LC record available at https://lccn.loc.gov/2019034447
LC ebook record available at https://lccn.loc.gov/2019034448

Visit the Taylor & Francis Web site at
http://www.taylorandfrancis.com

and the CRC Press Web site at
http://www.crcpress.com

CONTENTS

1

VENTRICULOMEGALY

The lateral ventricles should be measured at the routine mid-trimester scan in the axial plane at the level of the cavum septi pellucidi, with the calipers aligned with the internal borders of the medial and lateral walls of the ventricle; this should be at the level of the glomus of the choroid plexus. Fetal ventriculomegaly is characterized by a dilatation of the lateral ventricles, with or without dilatation of the third or fourth ventricles. There is no internationally agreed upon terminology, but Table 1.1 shows two systems used. It can affect one (unilateral) or both ventricles (bilateral).

When mild or moderate, it may be due to normal variation, but it also represents a common endpoint of various pathologic processes. As the outcome and prognosis depend on the underlying cause, investigations are aimed at determining this.

Apart from the underlying etiology and the presence of associated structural/chromosomal anomalies, post-natal outcome depends on the progression of ventricular dilatation. In isolated abnormality (absence of pathology and progression), the outlook for mild ventriculomegaly (<15 mm) is good with >95% of babies having normal neurodevelopment.

Associated major anomalies (cranial and extracranial) can be present in 50% of fetuses with VM, of which the most common are agenesis of the corpus callosum, posterior fossa malformations, and open spina bifida. The rate of associated anomalies in severe VM is higher than in mild VM.

Investigations needed

The prognosis is highly dependent on:

- Other fetal anomalies
- The cause of the ventriculomegaly
- Progression of the ventriculomegaly

Table 1.1 *Different classifications of ventriculomegaly used in the literature*

Normal measurement: <10 mm	Normal measurement: <10 mm
Mild ventriculomegaly: 10–12 mm	Mild ventriculomegaly: 10–15 mm
Moderate ventriculomegaly: 12–15 mm	
Severe ventriculomegaly: >15 mm	Severe ventriculomegaly: >15 mm

Investigations are therefore centered around these issues:

- Optimal imaging is needed: undertake (or refer for) detailed multiplanar neurosonography; transvaginal scanning is helpful. This should include assessment of:
  - The entire ventricular system
  - The periventricular zone/signs of hemorrhage
  - The pericerebral spaces and cortical fissures
- Consider fetal MRI.
- Review nuchal translucency and any previous chromosomal anomaly screening or prenatal diagnosis results.
- Consider karyotype by amniocentesis.
- Maternal serology for toxoplasma/CMV infection.
- Platelet group of parents to look for alloimmune thrombocytopenia should be considered if there is any possibility there could be intracranial bleeding.
- Follow up with further scans in the third trimester to assess for progression: It is important to explain to parents that prenatal imaging cannot completely rule out associated anomalies and that some may become evident only later in pregnancy or even at birth. The rate of associated anomalies detected only at follow-up scan is around 7%; progression of ventricular dilatation can occur in about 16% of cases.

Bibliography

Carta S, Kaelin Agten A, Belcaro C, Bhide A. Outcome of fetuses with prenatal diagnosis of isolated severe bilateral ventriculomegaly: Systematic review and meta-analysis. *Ultrasound Obstet Gynecol.* 2018 Aug; 52(2): 165–73.

Garel C, Luton D, Oury JF et al. Ventricular dilatations. *Childs Nerv Syst.* 2003; 19: 517–23.

International Society of Ultrasound in Obstetrics and Gynecology. Sonographic examination of the fetal central nervous system: Guidelines for performing the "basic examination" and the "fetal neurosonogram." *Ultrasound Obstet Gynecol.* 2007; 29: 109–16.

Melchiorre K, Bhide A, Gika AD et al. Counseling in isolated mild fetal ventriculomegaly. *Ultrasound Obstet Gynecol.* 2009; 34: 212–24.

Pagani G, Thilaganathan B, Prefumo F. Neurodevelopmental outcome in isolated mild fetal ventriculomegaly: Systematic review and meta-analysis. *Ultrasound Obstet Gynecol.* 2014; 44: 254–60.

Rossi AC, Prefumo F. Additional value of fetal magnetic resonance imaging in the prenatal diagnosis of central nervous system anomalies: A systematic review of the literature. *Ultrasound Obstet Gynecol.* 2014; 44: 388–93.

Scala C, Familiari A, Pinas A et al. Perinatal and long-term outcome in fetuses diagnosed with isolated unilateral ventriculomegaly: Systematic review and meta-analysis. *Ultrasound Obstet Gynecol.* 2016 Apr 19.

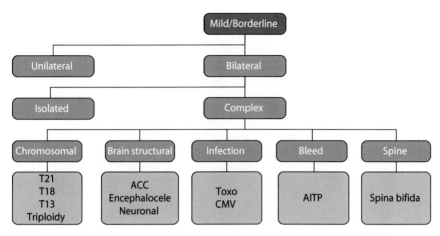

Algorithm 1.1 *Classifications of mild/borderline ventriculomegaly.*

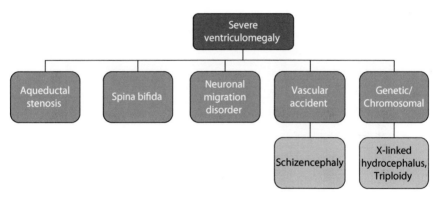

Algorithm 1.2 *Classifications of severe ventriculomegaly.*

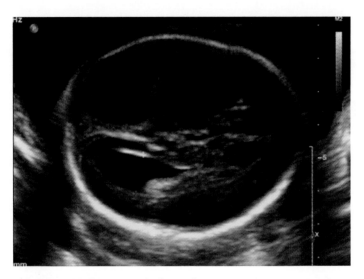

Figure 1.1 *Moderate ventriculomegaly.*

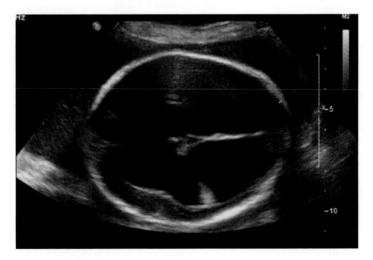

Figure 1.2 *Severe ventriculomegaly.*

2

INTRACRANIAL CYSTS

Many cystic structures in the fetal brain are not true cysts but can be pseudocysts. Distinguishing between the two can lead you to the diagnosis. True brain cysts have a capsule, regular margins, and may have a pressure effect. In contrast, pseudocysts have no capsule, irregular margins, and no compression effect.

Choroid plexus cysts are collections of the cerebrospinal fluid (CSF) due to blockage of the glands in the choroid plexus and seen in 1%–3% of fetuses at the time of the anomaly scan. They are associated with an increase in the risk of trisomy 18 (Edwards syndrome), however, they are rarely an isolated finding in this condition. Assess any prior screening for chromosomal anomalies including non-invasive prenatal screening using maternal cell-free DNA, nuchal translucency at 11–14 weeks, and check the maternal age. The association of choroid plexus cysts with trisomy 18 loses significance in women with previous low-risk screening. If the brain appears otherwise entirely normal, and if the cysts are not very large, they are harmless and almost always disappear later in the pregnancy. Reassurance can be offered and no further follow-up is necessary.

Arachnoid cysts are rare cysts arising from the arachnoid and contain cerebrospinal fluid. They do not communicate with the ventricular system. They are most often isolated, regular, and non-midline. The size can be very variable. Midline shift of the brain may be seen due to pressure effects. If they are isolated, the outlook is usually good, unless the size is very large.

The interhemispheric "cyst" is a misnomer as it is usually a pseudocyst. There is ultrasound appearance of a cystic structure in the midline. This is due to the deficiency in the roof of the third ventricle as a result of agenesis of the corpus callosum (see Chapter 3).

The aneurysm of vein of Galen is a rare malformation of the posterior cranial fossa. Vein of Galen is not a cyst, but rather a cranial venous sinus, which undergoes massive dilatation. Color flow mapping will show presence of moving blood. It can lead to a cardiac strain as evidenced by cardiac enlargement and increased pulsatility of the ductus venosus blood flow. In severe cases, hydrops fetalis can result.

Porencephalic cysts are destructive (clastic) lesions—they commonly communicate with the ventricle due to destruction of white matter. They are often due to brain hemorrhage and do not show a mass effect.

Cocaine use is associated with transient but intense vasospasm in blood vessels, including those supplying the brain. The malformations arising as a result of cocaine use defy any pattern.

Venous malformation is a recently described rare malformation in the posterior cranial fossa. The venous malformation can contain a blood clot or very slow flow rates, so there is no flow signal evident on color flow mapping. The limited available information suggests the outlook to be guarded due to pressure effects on the developing brain.

Cystic structures in the posterior fossa include:

- Enlarged cisterna magna when it is >10 mm in the transverse cerebellar view. Detailed ultrasound is needed to demonstrate this is isolated and that the cerebellum and vermis are normal. It can be associated with ventriculomegaly, but if it remains isolated and does not progress, prognosis is generally good.
- Blake's pouch cysts represent a communication between the 4th ventricle into the cisterna magna and appear as a unilocular cyst without any Doppler flow. Careful assessment is mandatory to ensure the remainder of the brain—in particular cerebellum and vermis—are normal. This is usually isolated, and most will resolve spontaneously.
- In Dandy-Walker malformation there is dilation of the fourth ventricle in the posterior fossa and that extends into the cisterna magna. The cerebellar vermis will be hypoplastic or absent. The condition is often associated with chromosomal abnormalities (mainly trisomy 18 and 13) or genetic syndromes. Coexisting abnormalities are very common, as is severe ventriculomegaly. The outlook is guarded.

Bibliography

Epelman M, Daneman A, Blaser SI et al. Differential diagnosis of intracranial cystic lesions at Head US: Correlation with CT and MR imaging. *RadioGraphics*. 2006; 26(1): 173–96.

Pilu G, Falco P, Perolo A et al. Differential diagnosis and outcome of fetal intracranial hypoechoic lesions: Report of 21 cases. *Ultrasound Obstet Gynecol*. 1997; 9: 229–36.

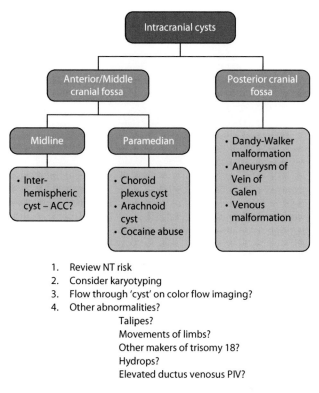

1. Review NT risk
2. Consider karyotyping
3. Flow through 'cyst' on color flow imaging?
4. Other abnormalities?
      Talipes?
      Movements of limbs?
      Other makers of trisomy 18?
      Hydrops?
      Elevated ductus venosus PIV?

Algorithm 2.1 *Classification of intracranial cysts and suggested work-up.*

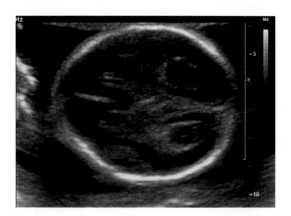

Figure 2.1 *Choroid plexus cyst.*

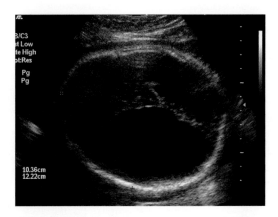

Figure 2.2 *Arachnoid cyst.*

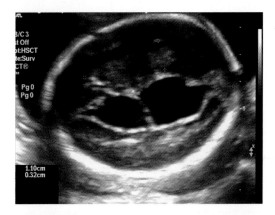

Figure 2.3 *Midline arachnoid (third ventricular) cyst.*

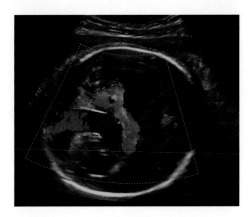

Figure 2.4 *Vein of Galen malformation.*

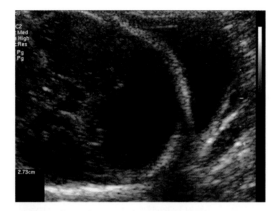

Figure 2.5 *Posterior fossa cyst.*

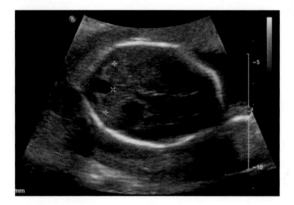

Figure 2.6 *Absent cerebellar vermis.*

3

AGENESIS OF CORPUS CALLOSUM

Corpus callosum is the largest bundle of fibers connecting the left and right cerebral hemispheres. Its absence is called agenesis of corpus callosum (ACC) and can be total or partial (usually posterior part missing). ACC has an estimated prevalence ranging from 2 per 10,000 in the general population to 200–600 per 10,000 in children with neurodevelopmental disabilities. Prenatal counseling can be very challenging given the vast spectrum of outcomes from normal to severe delay in motor and cognitive functions.

Suspecting ACC

Visualization of the corpus callosum is not part of routine second-trimester screening. ACC can however be suspected by indirect signs such as absent cavum septum pellucidum, ventriculomegaly, and midline lesions including lipomas and cysts. These indirect signs are inconsistent and not always encountered in fetuses with partial ACC.

Diagnosing ACC

Visualization of the corpus callosum on ultrasound requires additional views from the ones used for routine screening. Corpus callosum can usually be seen from 18 weeks in coronal and mid-sagittal views appearing as a thin anechoic space, bordered superiorly and inferiorly by echogenic lines. Visualization of the pericallosal artery in mid-sagittal view of the brain highlights the corpus callosum, running along the superior surface of the corpus callosum (absent in ACC).

Additional investigations

Karyotype/array comparative genomic hybridization (CGH): The rate of chromosomal anomalies in fetuses with complete and partial ACC is increased even in an isolated finding.

Fetal brain MRI: In cases of a prenatal diagnosis of isolated ACC, the risk of associated anomalies detected only at fetal MRI is about 10% in fetuses with ACC. The majority of additional anomalies detected at fetal MRI involve neuronal migration defects.

Prenatal counseling in isolated ACC

In about 70% of children with prenatal diagnosis of isolated ACC, normal neurodevelopmental outcome is reported. Delay in motor and cognitive functions, epilepsy, and social and language deficits are the most common symptoms reported in individuals with ACC. Furthermore, ACC has been linked with the occurrence of autism, schizophrenia, and attention-deficit disorders. Parents should be informed that prenatal imaging is not always able to differentiate between complex and isolated cases with additional post-natal findings diagnosed in about 5%–10% of cases of ACC.

Bibliography

D'Antonio F, Pagani G, Familiari A et al. Outcomes associated with isolated agenesis of the corpus callosum: A meta-analysis. *Pediatrics*. 2016; 138(3): e20160445.

Santo S, D'Antonio F, Homfray T, Rich P, Pilu G, Bhide A, Thilaganathan B, Papageorghiou T. Counseling in fetal medicine: Agenesis of the corpus callosum. *Ultrasound Obstet Gynecol*. 2012; 40: 513–21.

Youssef A, Ghi T, Pilu G. How to image the fetal corpus callosum. *Ultrasound Obstet Gynecol*. 2013; 42: 718–20.

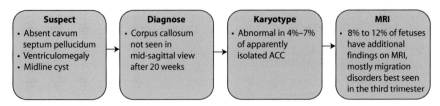

Suspect	**Diagnose**	**Karyotype**	**MRI**
• Absent cavum septum pellucidum • Ventriculomegaly • Midline cyst	• Corpus callosum not seen in mid-sagittal view after 20 weeks	• Abnormal in 4%–7% of apparently isolated ACC	• 8% to 12% of fetuses have additional findings on MRI, mostly migration disorders best seen in the third trimester

Algorithm 3.1 *Work-up of ACC.*

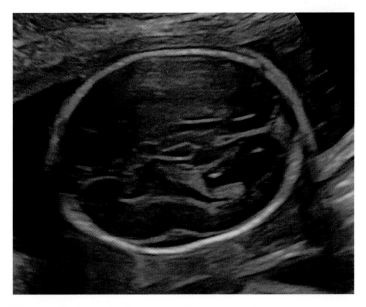

Figure 3.1 *Agenesis of corpus callosum, note absent cavum septum pellucidum.*

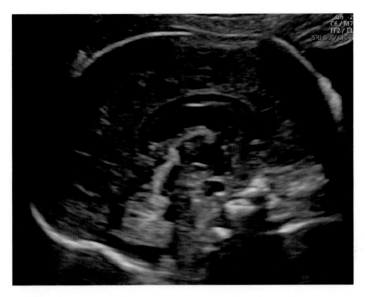

Figure 3.2 *Corpus callosum seen in mid-sagittal view.*

4

ABNORMAL SKULL SHAPE

During routine examination, the size and shape of the skull are assessed, as are the integrity of the skull and mineralization. Normally the skull has an oval shape and is continuously echogenic, with the sutures visible as narrow gaps.

Brachycephaly and dolichocephaly occur when the head is more rounded or elongated, respectively. This is most commonly a normal variant:

- In brachycephaly the head appears shorter and wider. This is most often due to normal variation but has also been associated with trisomy 21. Premature fusion of the coronal sutures can also be a cause; this is seen in Pfeiffer syndrome, where wide-set eyes, brachydactyly or syndactyly may also coexist.
- Dolichocephaly is frequently associated with pressure effects due to a fetal breech presentation or reduced amniotic fluid. In late gestation it can be due to premature fusion of the sagittal suture.

A lemon-shaped skull is a classic sign of an open neural tube defect. The lemon shape is most often seen in the middle third of pregnancy and can resolve in the third trimester. In open spina bifida it is associated with a banana-shaped cerebellum. "Lemon-like" skull without spina bifida has no clinical significance, but a very careful search of the spine is indicated before disregarding this finding (refer to Chapter 27).

A strawberry-shaped skull should raise the suspicion of trisomy 18 (Edwards syndrome). Check prior screening: maternal age is more likely to be advanced and the nuchal translucency may have been raised at 11–14 weeks. Early-onset growth restriction is often present, and the pregnancy may have been re-dated on an early scan. Other indicators of trisomy 18 may be present, such as choroid plexus cysts, micrognathia, congenital heart disease, exomphalos, and talipes equinovarus. Trigonocephaly, of similar appearance, is due to fusion of the metopic suture and can also be part of Jacobsen or Opitz C syndromes.

Cloverleaf- or trilobate-shaped skull can be associated with thanatophoric dysplasia, a lethal form of skeletal dysplasia (see Chapter 27). The finding may also be seen in Apert syndrome or Crouzon syndrome.

Encephalocele is associated with a defect of the skull. Posterior encephaloceles are much more common than at other sites. The size is variable, ranging from larger than the skull to very small—so as to easily be missed. One should also look for features of Meckel–Gruber syndrome (occipital encephalocele, polycystic kidneys, polydactyly), as it has autosomal recessive inheritance.

In some conditions the skull is very poorly mineralized and is easily deformed by the pressure of the ultrasound probe. This can be due to hypophosphatasia; in achondrogenesis, a lethal skeletal dysplasia, there is also severe shortening of the long bones.

Bibliography

Accardi MC, Lo Magno E, Ermito S et al. Echotomography of craniosynostosis: Review of literature. *J Prenat Med*. 2009 Apr; 3(2): 31–3.

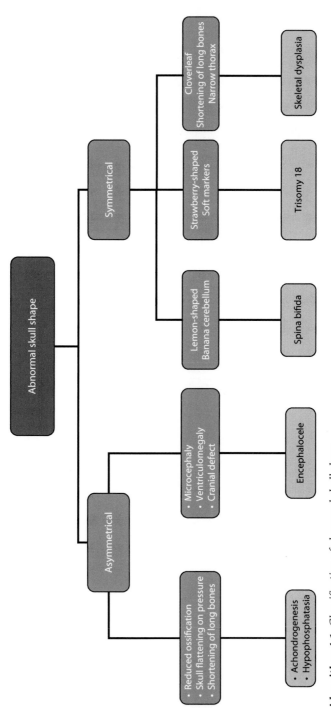

Algorithm 4.1 *Classification of abnormal skull shape.*

(a) (b)

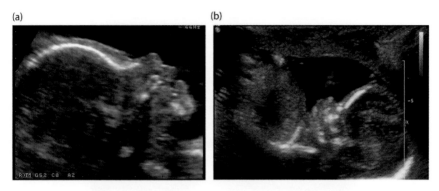

Figure 4.1 *(a) Normal mid-sagittal section of face. (b) Frontal bossing.*

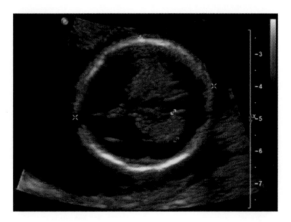

Figure 4.2 *Brachycephaly.*

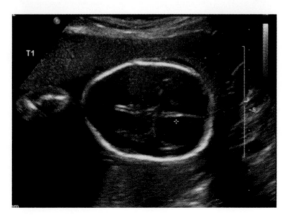

Figure 4.3 *Lemon-shaped head.*

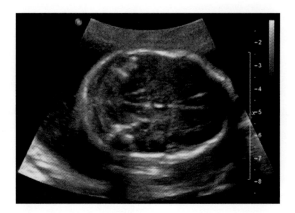

Figure 4.4 *Banana cerebellum.*

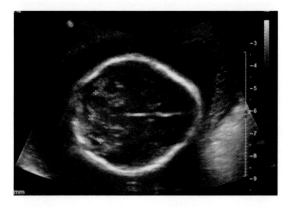

Figure 4.5 *Strawberry-shaped head.*

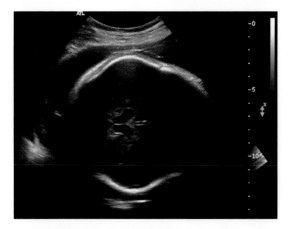

Figure 4.6 *Cloverleaf-shaped head.*

5

FACIAL CLEFTS

Facial clefts are usually isolated but may be associated with other medical conditions such as chromosomal abnormality, genetic syndromes, and a family history of facial clefts. Cleft lip is associated with a cleft palate in the majority of cases.

Ultrasound recognition involves obtaining a coronal surface view of the face showing lips and nostrils. The defect in the alveolar ridge is demonstrable on a transverse view. A profile view shows "pre-maxillary protrusion" in cases of bilateral cleft lip/alveolus. The palate is not normally visualized on ultrasound; however, a defect of the alveolar ridge can be demonstrated, and in most cases, is associated with a defect of the hard palate.

Pre-natal diagnosis of cleft palate without cleft lip/alveolus is extremely difficult. The use of "reverse face view" on 3-D ultrasound has been described to improve pre-natal identification of defects of the palate. The "equals sign" (a typical echo pattern of the normal uvula) could help in evaluation of the soft palate in the event of a cleft lip and palate. Visualization of the equals sign proves an intact palate. Absence of the equals sign indicates a cleft palate and should prompt further examination of the soft palate in a median sagittal section. Cleft palate can be confirmed when the soft palate cannot be visualized.

Careful examination of the fetal heart and brain structure is indicated. The threshold for referral for fetal echocardiography should be low.

Median and bilateral cleft lip/alveolus are associated with a higher risk of underlying chromosomal abnormality or midline structural abnormalities of the brain. Prenatal identification of associated genetic syndromes is also very difficult in the absence of past or family history. Facial cleft is a recognized feature of trisomy 13.

Trisomy 13 (Patau syndrome): Mother's age is likely to be advanced. The nuchal translucency may have been raised at 11–14 weeks. Cell-free DNA might have already been performed in the first trimester. Other indicators of trisomy 13 may be present; there may be CNS abnormalities such as ventriculomegaly or holoprosencephaly. Heart abnormalities are present in over 95% of fetuses. Polydactyly and rocker bottom feet may be seen.

Bibliography

James JN, Schlieder DW. Prenatal counseling, ultrasound diagnosis, and the role of maternal-fetal medicine of the cleft lip and palate patient. *Oral Maxillofac Surg Clin North Am.* 2016; 28: 145–51.
Wilhelm L, Borgers H. The "equals sign": A novel marker in the diagnosis of fetal isolated cleft palate. *Ultrasound Obstet Gynecol.* 2010; 36: 439–44.

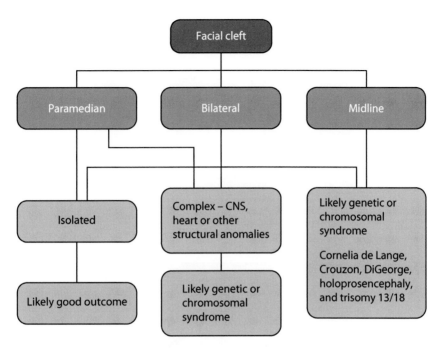

Algorithm 5.1 *Classification of facial clefts.*

(a)

(b)

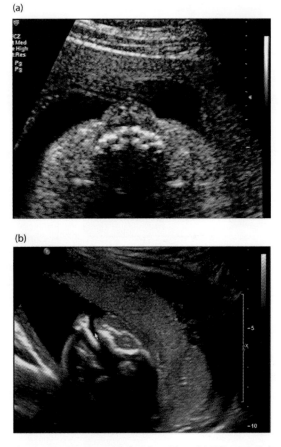

Figure 5.1 *(a) Normal alveolar ridge. (b) Bilateral cleft alveolus and primary palate.*

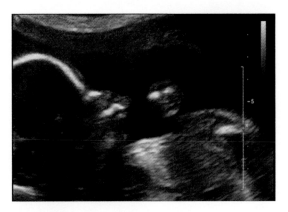

Figure 5.2 *Pre-maxillary protrusion.*

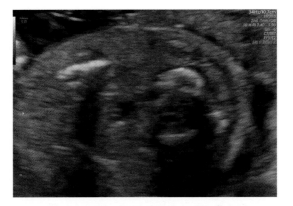

Figure 5.3 *The "equals sign."*

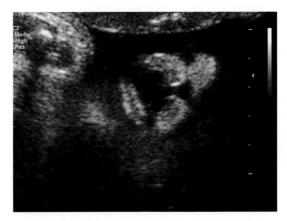

Figure 5.4 *Unilateral cleft lip.*

6

MICROGNATHIA

The chin is best visualized on profile view of the face. There is no definition for micrognathia, and the diagnosis is subjective. Unless severe, ultrasound prenatal diagnosis can be very difficult.

Goldenhar syndrome: Also known as "hemifacial microsomia," this is a birth defect involving first and second branchial arch derivatives. There is asymmetry between structures on the left as opposed to the right side of the face. In addition to craniofacial anomalies, there may be cardiac, vertebral, and central nervous system defects. Most cases are sporadic, but some show autosomal dominant inheritance.

Trisomy 13 (Patau syndrome): The mother's age is likely to be advanced. The nuchal translucency may have been raised at 11–14 weeks. Cell-free DNA might have already been performed in the first trimester. Other indicators of trisomy 13 may be present, such as ventriculomegaly, holoprosencephaly, polydactyly, rocker bottom feet, and cardiac abnormalities, in over 95% of fetuses.

Trisomy 18 (Edwards syndrome): The mother's age is likely to be advanced. The nuchal translucency may have been raised at 11–14 weeks. Cell-free DNA might have already been performed in the first trimester. Early-onset growth restriction is often present, and the pregnancy may have been re-dated on an early scan. Other indicators of trisomy 18 may be present—choroid plexus cysts, ventriculomegaly, clenched fists, congenital heart disease (often complex), exomphalos, single umbilical artery, and talipes equinovarus.

CHARGE association consists of a combination of choanal atresia, colobomas, heart abnormalities, growth restriction, and neurodevelopmental handicap. Many of these, apart from cardiac abnormalities, are very difficult to detect on prenatal ultrasound scan. Asymmetry of structures can sometimes be seen in CHARGE association. Although the inheritance is thought to be autosomal dominant, many cases are due to sporadic new mutations.

DiGeorge syndrome is also sometimes referred to as CATCH22 (cardiac abnormality/abnormal facies, T-cell deficit due to thymic hypoplasia, cleft palate, hypocalcemia due to hypoparathyroidism) resulting from 22q11 microdeletion. Disturbance of cervical neural crest migration into the derivatives of the pharyngeal arches and pouches can account for the phenotype. Most cases are sporadic and result from a deletion of chromosome 22q11.2. However, autosomal dominant inheritance is known. Mild to moderate learning difficulties are common.

Treacher–Collins syndrome is also called mandibulofacial dysostosis. The features include antimongoloid slant of the eyes, coloboma of the lid, micrognathia, cleft palate, microtia, hypoplastic zygomatic arches, and macrostomia. Apart from micrognathia, the other features are difficult to detect on pre-natal ultrasound. This is an autosomal dominant disorder with variable expression.

Smith–Lemli–Opitz Syndrome (SLOS): A deficiency of 7-dehydrocholesterol reductase is a causative factor of the SLO syndrome. There is evidence of pre-natal onset of growth restriction. Ambiguous genitals and sex reversal in male fetuses are seen. Polydactyly and microcephaly are often present. Mental retardation is present. Inheritance is autosomal recessive.

Bibliography

Paladini D. Fetal micrognathia: Almost always an ominous finding. *Ultrasound Obstet Gynecol.* 2010; 35: 377–84.

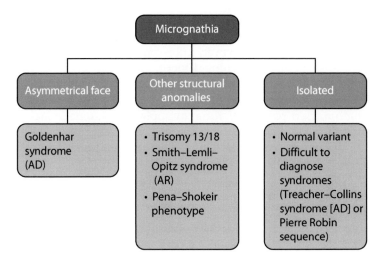

Algorithm 6.1 *Classification of micrognathia.*

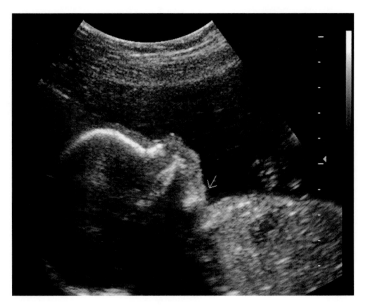

Figure 6.1 *Micrognathia.*

7

NASAL BONE

The association of nasal bone hypoplasia and trisomy 21 is well established. There are ultrasound studies in low- and high-risk populations, as well as histopathological studies in fetuses with Down syndrome, which have consistently confirmed this association. It is established that 50%–60% of fetuses with Down syndrome will have absent/hypoplastic nasal bones at 11–14 weeks on ultrasound scanning and also on autopsy studies. However, nasal bones can be absent in chromosomally normal fetuses as well. In a large population-based study, nasal bone was found to be absent at 11–14 weeks in 0.5% of normal fetuses (this figure varies with parental ethnicity).

Advanced maternal age, increased nuchal translucency, abnormal serum biochemistry, and abnormalities or soft markers seen on ultrasound scans are the factors to be considered in determining the *a priori* risk and would define a "high-risk" population. Absence of nasal bones would significantly increase the chance of underlying trisomy 21, and an invasive test should be considered. On the other hand, prevalence of trisomy 21 in the low-risk population is low. Failure to visualize the fetal nasal bones could easily be a variation of normal. The significance of nasal bone as a screening marker for trisomy 21 is questionable following the introduction of cell-free DNA testing.

Bibliography

Cicero S, Curcio P, Papageorghiou A, Sonek J, Nicolaides K. Absence of nasal bone in fetuses with trisomy 21 at 11–14 weeks of gestation: An observational study. *Lancet.* 2001; 358(9294): 1665–7.

Prefumo F, Sairam S, Bhide A, Thilaganathan B. First-trimester nuchal translucency, nasal bones, and trisomy 21 in selected and unselected populations. *Am J Obstetrics and Gynecology* 2006; 194: 828–33.

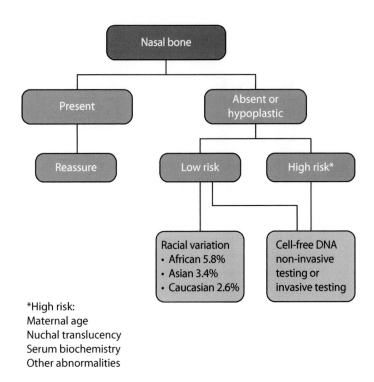

*High risk:
Maternal age
Nuchal translucency
Serum biochemistry
Other abnormalities

Algorithm 7.1 *Classification of nasal bone.*

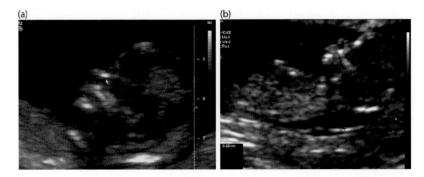

Figure 7.1 *(a) First-trimester nasal bones. (b) First-trimester absent nasal bones.*

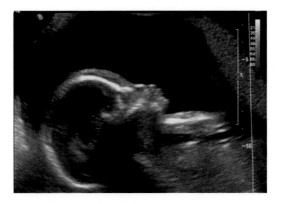

Figure 7.2 *Second-trimester hypoplastic nasal bone.*

8

HYPERTELORISM

Hypertelorism refers to an interocular distance above the 95th percentile. Causes of hypertelorism include mechanical causes such as premature fusion of the skull bones or a cleft. Genetic syndromes such as craniofrontonasal dysplasia, Apert syndrome, and Crouzon syndrome can have hypertelorism as part of their features. Mild hypertelorism can also be present as an isolated finding with no clinical consequences.

The inner and outer interocular distances are not routinely measured during second-trimester ultrasound. However, in the presence of other fetal anomalies, especially facial clefts, abnormal skull shape, micrognathia, and brain defects, a detailed study of the face can contribute to the diagnosis of an underlying condition. Surgical correction of hypertelorism is nowadays available but the outcome is mostly dictated by the underlying condition.

Bibliography

Ondeck CL, Pretorius D, McCaulley J, Kinori M, Maloney T, Hull A, Robbins SL. Ultrasonographic prenatal imaging of fetal ocular and orbital abnormalities. *Surv Ophthalmol.* 2018; 63: 745–753.

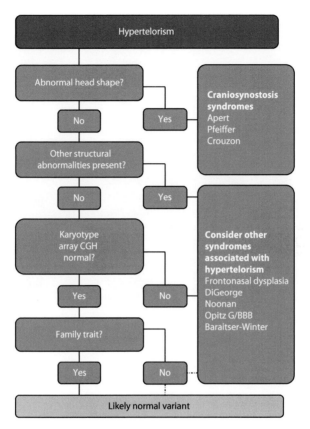

Algorithm 8.1 *Classification of hypertelorism.*

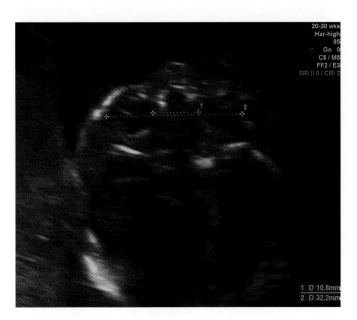

Figure 8.1 *Hypertelorism.*

9

CHEST TUMORS

The majority of fetal chest tumors are benign and tend to be identified in the second trimester. In the absence of fetal hydrops, they have a favorable prognosis. They are identified as echogenic lesions or mixed lesions with anechoic lesions interspersed within the echogenic areas.

The vast majority of chest lesions tend to be unilateral and in many cases present with a shift of the mediastinum easily spotted with the heart axis being deviated to one side. A predominantly cystic lesion is usually a congenital cystic adenomatoid malformation (CCAM) of the macrocystic variety. These tend to be isolated lesions in the fetus and may very occasionally need to be drained in order to avoid the consequence of cardiac compression. A predominantly echogenic lesion should be approached with the differential diagnoses of CCAM, pulmonary sequestration, or temporary bronchial obstruction. The presence of systemic arterial supply from the thoracic or abdominal dorsal aorta would suggest the diagnosis of sequestration. Most of the lesions are found to have both CCAM and sequestration on histopathological examination. It is recommended to monitor these pregnancies serially in order to exclude the development of fetal hydrops. The majority of bronchial obstruction and CCAM, however, regress spontaneously so much so that as the pregnancy advances, the lesions are difficult to identify on scan. In any case, post-natal follow-up is recommended with CT scans of the chest, as the surgeons might consider removing any residual lesions in the chest.

The presence of unilateral lesion with mixed echoes should raise the suspicion of a congenital diaphragmatic hernia (CDH), especially with mediastinal deviation and the lack of a stomach bubble in the normal position. This should also prompt a thorough search for other markers and abnormalities as there is a high risk of underlying chromosomal and structural abnormalities. A detailed fetal echocardiography is necessary to rule out possible associated cardiac abnormalities. In general, an isolated left-sided diaphragmatic hernia tends to be better than the right-sided one involving the liver. Additional extracardiac malformations would dictate a poorer prognosis.

The presence of bilateral chest lesions suggests either bilateral CCAM or a congenital high airway obstruction syndrome (CHAOS). This may have additional features such as an inverted dome of the fetal diaphragm and dilated airways. A significant proportion also present with ascites owing to obstruction to the venous return to the heart. In addition to planning serial scans to assess any cardiac compromise, these fetuses need to be delivered in tertiary referral centers in order to assess the need for surgical intervention soon after birth.

Midline chest lesions in the fetus may be enteric, thymic, or pericardial in origin. Enteric or bronchogenic midline tumors are usually cystic and tend to be benign. Unless they are huge and compress the cardiac structures, they tend to be associated with a good outcome. Pericardial tumors are usually teratomas and may present initially as pericardial effusions. Depending on their exact site on the pericardial surface, they may cause rhythm disturbances and are potentially dangerous. The presence of pericardial effusion should prompt a thorough search for such tumors. Additionally, pericardiocentesis may be life-saving for the fetus and would be required to promote normal growth and development of the fetal lungs.

Bibliography

Davenport M, Warne SA, Cacciaguerra S, Patel S, Greenough A, Nicolaides K. Current outcome of antenatally diagnosed cystic lung disease. *J Pediatr Surg.* 2004; 39(4): 549–56.

Gajewska-Knapik K, Impey L. Congenital lung lesions: Prenatal diagnosis and intervention. *Semin Pediatr Surg.* 2015; 24: 156–9.

Lim FY, Crombleholme TM, Hedrick HL, Flake AW, Johnson MP, Howell LJ, Adzick NS. Congenital high airway obstruction syndrome: Natural history and management. *J Pediatr Surg.* 2003; 38(6): 940–5.

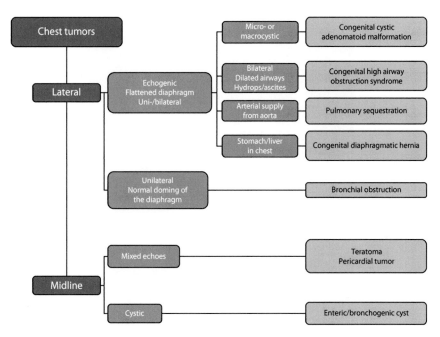

Algorithm 9.1 *Differential classification of chest tumors.*

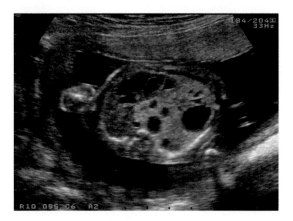

Figure 9.1 *Macrocystic lung lesion.*

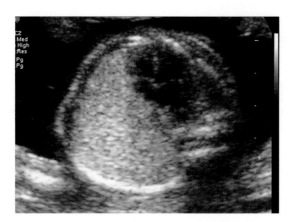

Figure 9.2 *Microcystic lung lesion.*

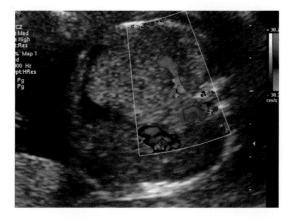

Figure 9.3 *Pulmonary sequestration.*

10

CHEST FLUID

Fluid in the fetal chest is seen not uncommonly during the anomaly scan and occasionally during routine growth scans scheduled for other indications. The fluid may be seen as a cystic collection or as pleural or pericardial effusion. Cystic collections in the lungs or mediastinum need to be dealt with as chest tumors. Pleural effusion is seen as fluid collection around the compressed lung. Pleural or pericardial effusions may occur simultaneously in some conditions but usually tend to be independent of each other.

Pleural effusion may present as part of a generalized immune or non-immune fetal hydrops, accompanying a structural anomaly or, more rarely, an isolated finding. Most primary pleural effusions become chylous (with the onset of post-natal feeding) and occur either due to excessive production or reduced reabsorption of lymphatic fluid. A thorough search should be made to identify any possible associated structural abnormality in the fetus and in the placenta. Presence of fetal growth abnormalities may suggest an underlying congenital viral infection. The presence of skin edema with or without ascites should prompt a search both in the history and on scan for conditions such as red cell isoimmunization, parvovirus infection, and possible A-V malformations. Placental chorioangioma is sometimes forgotten in these situations, but forms an important treatable cause for the hyperdynamic circulation and cardiac failure.

Even in the absence of any other chromosomal marker, pleural effusion carries a 10% risk for chromosomal abnormalities, and therefore a pre-natal diagnosis should be offered to the couple. In many cases, the underlying etiology remains undetected even after birth. However, the effusion may still pose a problem by hindering the normal lung development depending on the gestational age of appearance and by causing cardiac compression. Several authors recommend thoracoamniotic shunting to relieve the thoracic pressure and to promote lung development. The management of pleural effusion should include a complete workup, as in any non-immune hydrops.

Prenatal sonographic identification of a small rim of pericardial fluid is a normal finding. Pericardial effusion is a subjective diagnosis unless the fluid collection is obviously large. It may manifest as an isolated finding or as a manifestation of an underlying pericardial tumor, fetal arrhythmia/cardiac structural abnormality, or rarely with a ventricular or atrial aneurysm or diverticulum. The clinical significance of isolated pericardial effusion has not been understood. The suspicion of a pericardial effusion warrants detailed echocardiography.

Bibliography

Santolaya-Forgas J. How do we counsel patients carrying a fetus with pleural effusions? *Ultrasound Obstet Gynecol.* 2001; 18(4): 305–8.

Slesnick TC, Ayres NA, Altman CA, Bezold LI, Eidem BW, Fraley JK, Kung GC, McMahon CJ, Pignatelli RH, Kovalchin JP. Characteristics and outcomes of fetuses with pericardial effusions. *Am J Cardiol.* 2005; 96(4): 599–601.

Yinon Y, Kelly E, Ryan G. Fetal pleural effusions. *Best Pract Res Clin Obstet Gynaecol.* 2008; 22: 77–96.

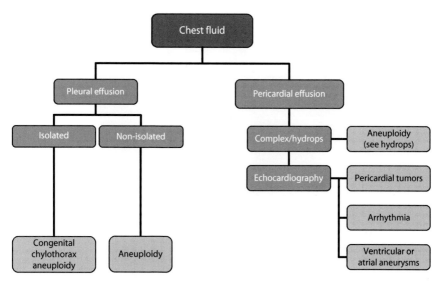

Algorithm 10.1 *Classification of chest fluid.*

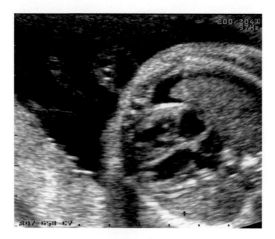

Figure 10.1 *Mild pleural effusion.*

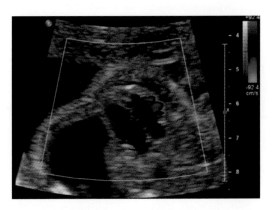

Figure 10.2 *Moderate pleural effusion and mediastinal shift.*

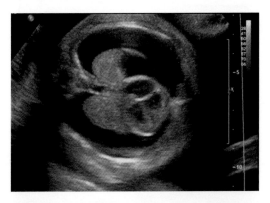

Figure 10.3 *Severe pleural effusion and fetal hydrops.*

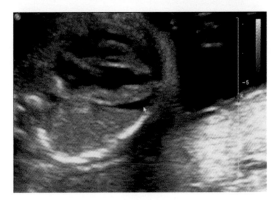

Figure 10.4 *Pericardial effusion.*

11

RIGHT-SIDED AORTIC ARCH

A right-sided aortic arch (RAA) is characterized by abnormal laterality and course of the aorta and brachiocephalic vessels. It courses abnormally to the right side of the trachea, as opposed to the normal left-sided aortic arch (LAA). In view of the association with other cardiac abnormalities, extracardiac abnormalities (such as thymus agenesis, isolated defects in the palate, and esophageal atresia), and chromosomal defects (such as DiGeorge/22q11.2 deletion), detailed ultrasound assessment, fetal echo, and pre-natal diagnosis are recommended.

Variations of aortic laterality and branching pattern are thought to be the result of an abnormal regression of the primordial paired aortic arches during embryonic life. Normal regression leads to an LAA, left-sided arterial duct (AD), and the usual branching pattern of brachiocephalic vessels represented by the right innominate artery, followed by the left common carotid and left subclavian arteries (LSA), respectively. RAA may have a mirror-image branching pattern, but an aberrant origin of the LSA (ALSA) is common.

RAA can also result in the formation of a vascular ring, which may be asymptomatic, but could also result in symptoms of compression, such as dysphagia, stridor, wheeze, and recurrent upper respiratory tract infections. The position of the AD and the course of the LSA should be noted in order to identify if a vascular ring is present, as this will require longer follow-up after birth. Special attention should also be given to the possibility of there being a double aortic arch.

Bibliography

Achiron R, Rotstein Z, Heggesh J et al. Anomalies of the fetal aortic arch: A novel sonographic approach to in-utero diagnosis. *Ultrasound Obstet Gynecol*. 2002; 20: 553–7.

D'Antonio F, Khalil A, Zidere V, Carvalho JS. Fetuses with right aortic arch: A multicenter cohort study and meta-analysis. *Ultrasound Obstet Gynecol*. 2016 Apr; 47(4): 423–32.

12

ABERRANT RIGHT SUBCLAVIAN ARTERY

Aberrant right subclavian artery (ARSA) can be demonstrated in the three vessels and trachea view as a vessel leading from the junction of the aortic arch and the ductus arteriosus, behind the trachea, and toward the right clavicle and shoulder. It is sought by lowering the color Doppler velocity range to 10–15 cm/s. In this plane, it is important not to confuse ARSA with the azygos vein, which appears to course in the direction of the superior vena cava. When ARSA is suspected, its presence can be confirmed by demonstrating arterial flow on pulsed Doppler. If the right subclavian artery has a normal origin, it is found in a plane of the transverse aortic arch that is more cranial than the three vessels and trachea view, and it courses ventrally from the trachea.

ARSA is more frequent in trisomy 21 fetuses and in fetuses with other chromosomal aberrations, including microdeletion 22q11. Therefore, the finding of ARSA during prenatal ultrasound scan should prompt a detailed anomaly scan by a fetal medicine specialist, referral to fetal echo, and prenatal diagnosis of aneuploidy. ARSA occasionally causes pressure on the esophagus and may cause dysphagia.

Bibliography

Chaoui R, Rake A, Heling KS. Aortic arch with four vessels: Aberrant right subclavian artery. *Ultrasound Obstet Gynecol*. 2008 Jan; 31(1): 115–7.

De León-Luis J, Gámez F, Bravo C et al. Second-trimester fetal aberrant right subclavian artery: Original study, systematic review and meta-analysis of performance in detection of Down syndrome. *Ultrasound Obstet Gynecol*. 2014 Aug; 44(2): 147–53.

13

DEXTROCARDIA

Fetal dextrocardia is a condition in which the major axis of the heart points to the right. The term dextrocardia describes only the position of the cardiac axis and conveys no information regarding chamber organization and structural anatomy of the heart.

Dextrocardia should be distinguished from dextroposition, in which the heart is shifted into the right chest as a consequence of pathological states involving the diaphragm, lung, pleura, or other adjoining tissues. The appearance of a smaller right side in the fetal chest should raise the suspicion of hypoplasia of the right lung with anomalous pulmonary venous drainage as in Scimitar syndrome.

The presence of the stomach bubble with/without bowel in the chest indicates a left-sided diaphragmatic hernia. This finding should prompt a thorough search for other markers of chromosomal abnormalities.

Hyperechoic areas may be seen occupying all or part of the lung field, suggesting a high airway obstruction or congenital cystic adenomatoid malformation (CCAM). The presence of cystic spaces should also raise the possibility of pulmonary sequestration or the mixed type of CCAM. The former is confirmed by the presence of arterial supply from the dorsal aorta with venous return which may be normal or anomalous. A clear collection of pleural fluid should raise the possibility of underlying chromosomal disorders, in addition to searching for other causes of cardiac decompensation.

True dextrocardia tends to be associated with situs abnormalities. Situs, by definition, relates to the fetal left-right orientation and preponderance of derivatives of left- or right-sided embryological elements. Situs can be assessed at various levels, namely abdominal, atrial, and pulmonary levels, and is usually similar at all levels. Situs solitus refers to usual arrangement of left- and right-sided structures with the dorsal aorta in the left side of the fetal abdomen and the IVC on the right. The atrial situs is indicated by the characteristic shape of the atrial appendages (broad in the right and digit-like on the left) and may be either left- or right-sided or ambiguous.

It is quite difficult to assess atrial situs in a fetus with ante-natal ultrasound and often not necessary for a diagnosis. As a routine, sonographers should get into the habit of assessing fetal right and left and then check the position of the abdominal aorta and IVC along with the stomach prior to assessing the fetal heart. This gives indications to the fetal situs in the majority of cases. Any variation from the normal warrants detailed fetal echo even in the absence of dextrocardia. With dextrocardia, the likelihood of structural cardiac abnormalities increases, and therefore a referral for fetal echo should be made. In the presence of situs inversus and dextrocardia with a structurally normal heart, the child will still need post-natal follow-up for other associated conditions such as Kartagener's syndrome (ciliary dyskinesia).

Bibliography

Bernasconi A, Azancot A, Simpson JM et al. Fetal dextrocardia: Diagnosis and outcome in two tertiary centres. *Heart.* 2005; 91: 1590–94.

Holzmann D, Ott PM, Felix H. Diagnostic approach to primary ciliary dyskinesia: A review. *Eur J Pediatr.* 2000; 159(1–2): 95–8.

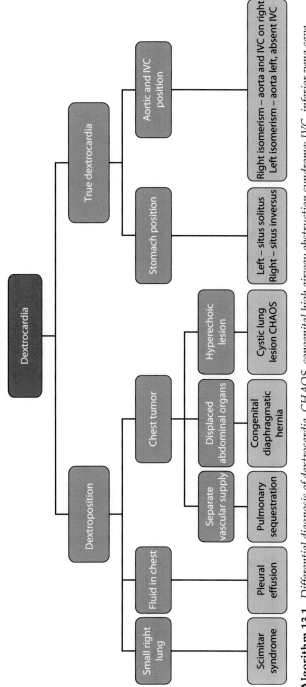

Algorithm 13.1 *Differential diagnosis of dextrocardia. CHAOS, congenital high airway obstruction syndrome; IVC, inferior vena cava.*

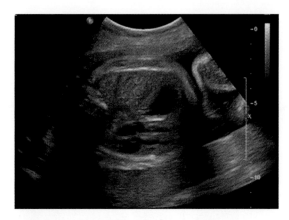

Figure 13.1 *Congenital diaphragmatic hernia.*

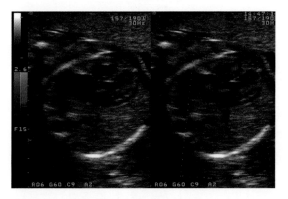

Figure 13.2 *Dextrocardia.*

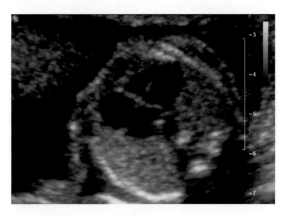

Figure 13.3 *Axis deviation.*

14

ABNORMAL
FOUR-CHAMBER VIEW

In routine screening of the fetal heart, one should ideally be able to extend views to check the outflow tracts and use color Doppler to assess the fetal heart thoroughly. However, given time constraints for a routine scan, this chapter confines itself to just the four-chamber view.

The following is a checklist for scanning the fetal heart:

1. Check abdominal situs. This is imperative to understand the left and right of the fetus and ensure that the fetal heart and stomach are on the fetal left side.
2. The fetal heart points to the left side with the majority of the heart lying in the left chest.
3. The heart occupies a third of the chest area.
4. There are four chambers with symmetrical ventricles and atria.
5. The moderator band is identified and indicates the right ventricle.
6. There are two A-V valves opening and closing (cineloop helps) and their point of attachment to the interventricular septum shows an offset with the tricuspid valve being closer to the apex when compared to the mitral valve.
7. The septum is intact (preferably checked with the septum horizontally oriented).

Further examinations should check the outflow tracts and ensure crossover. Much of this can be assessed using the three-vessel view. Any suspicious variations in any of these features should prompt a referral for detailed fetal echocardiography.

Situs abnormalities and cardiac axis deviation are discussed in Chapter 13.

Cardiomegaly by itself is an indicator for detailed fetal echocardiography and detailed fetal assessment of the hemodynamic state in the fetus. It is usually secondary to some other fetal pathology including growth restriction, hyperdynamic circulatory states such as anemia (parvovirus, red cell isoimmunization), A-V malformations in the fetus, placental chorioangioma, and occasionally fetal brady or tachyarrhythmias. Primary causes include major cardiac structural abnormalities and will need detailed assessment that is beyond the scope of this chapter. Needless to say, a suspicion of cardiomegaly warrants a detailed fetal echocardiography.

Asymmetry of the cardiac chambers usually reflects a structural problem in the A-V or outflow tract valves. Rare causes include anomalous venous drainage of the pulmonary veins where the drainage is into the right side of the heart rather than the left side of the heart in one or more veins.

The loss of a normal offset between the A-V valves suggests the presence of an A-V canal defect—called the A-V septal defect—and this is associated with a 50%–60% risk of underlying chromosomal abnormalities. This should prompt a thorough search for other markers for chromosomal abnormalities. A significant proportion of these will also have situs abnormalities (see Chapter 13).

Bibliography

Bolnick AD, Zelop CM, Milewski B et al. Use of the mitral valve-tricuspid valve distance as a marker of fetal endocardial cushion defects. *Am J Obstet Gynecol.* 2004; 191(4): 1483–5.

Del Bianco A, Russo S, Lacerenza N et al. Four chamber view plus three-vessel and trachea view for a complete evaluation of the fetal heart during the second trimester. *J Perinat Med.* 2006; 34(4): 309–12.

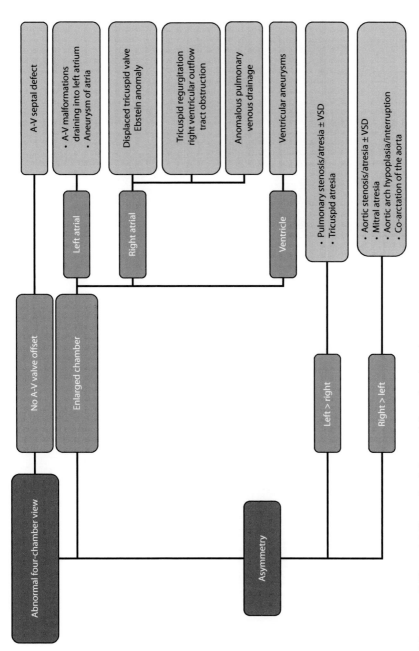

Algorithm 14.1 *Differential diagnosis of abnormal four-chamber view.*

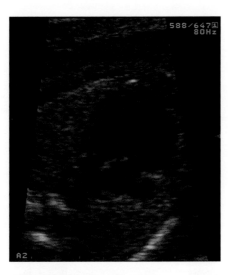

Figure 14.1 *Ventricular asymmetry.*

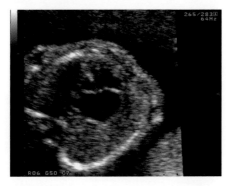

Figure 14.2 *Ventricular septal defect.*

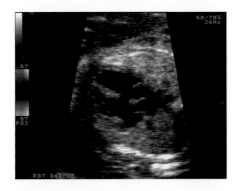

Figure 14.3 *Color Doppler demonstration of ventriculoseptal defect.*

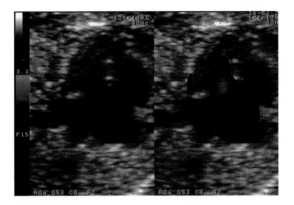

Figure 14.4 *Atrio-ventriculoseptal defect.*

15

ABNORMAL CARDIAC RHYTHM

Normal fetal heart rate is between 110 and 160 bpm. Periods of transient bradycardia or tachycardia are common and are of no clinical significance. When a fetal cardiac arrhythmia is diagnosed, extracardiac causes of tachycardia such as maternal medication (salbutamol, terbutaline), maternal pyrexia, and hyperthyroidism must first be excluded.

Fetal structural abnormality

Once extracardiac causes of fetal arrhythmia have been excluded, the fetal heart should be carefully examined to exclude structural abnormalities. Fetal arrhythmias can be part of complex structural heart conditions and in these cases, prognosis will be mostly determined by the underlying condition.

Fetal cardiac functional defects

Fetal arrhythmias can also present with some degree of heart failure, and it is important to document the presence or absence of cardiomegaly, atrioventricular valve regurgitation, pericardial effusion, and hydrops.

Ectopic beats

Ectopic beats are the most common form of fetal arrhythmia and usually present in the third trimester. Ectopic beats are caused by an extra beat arising prematurely and outside the natural pacemaker. They are of no clinical relevance, are not a sign of fetal distress, and do not need any form of treatment. The irregular rhythm due to ectopic beats tends to spontaneously resolve near term and does not need specific post-natal follow-up. In the rare case of bigeminy or very frequent ectopic beats, there is a risk of the fetus developing a persistent tachyarrhythmia, and therefore weekly monitoring of the fetal heart rate is recommended.

Fetal tachyarrhythmia

Fetal tachyarrhythmia (e.g., SVT with 1:1 AV conduction and atrial flutter) can be treated in utero, with digoxin, sotalol, or flecainide, depending on type of arrhythmia, presence of hydrops, gestational age, and physician's preference. In view of the pro-arrhythmic risk for the mother, an ECG should be arranged before and during treatment.

Fetal bradycardias

Fetal bradycardias secondary to complete heart block do not have specific in-utero treatment, but close monitoring to optimize time of delivery and post-natal assessment for pacemaker implantation can have a major impact on outcome. Parental 12-lead ECG and maternal auto-antibody status (anti-Ro and anti-La) should be obtained.

Bibliography

Bravo-Valenzuela NJ, Rocha LA, Machado Nardozza LM et al. Fetal cardiac arrhythmias: Current evidence. *Ann Pediatr Cardiol.* 2018; 11: 148–63.

Carvalho JS, Fetal dysrhythmias. *Best Pract Res Clin Obstet Gynaecol.* https://doi.org/10.1016/j.bpobgyn.2019.01.002.

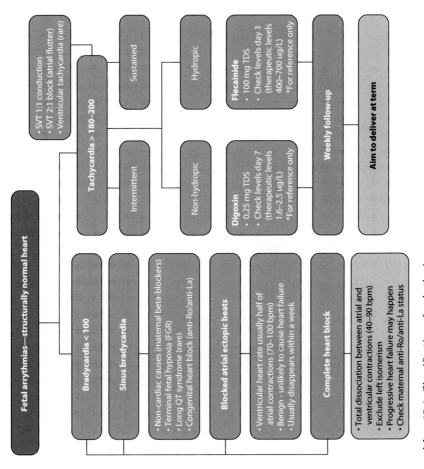

Algorithm 15.1 *Classification of arrhythmias.*

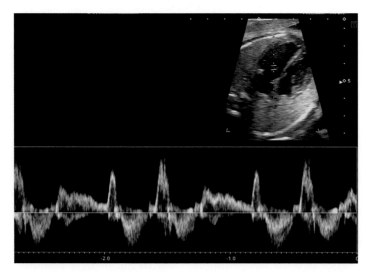

Figure 15.1 *Ectopic beats.*

16

ABDOMINAL WALL DEFECT

The physiological gut herniation into the umbilical sac is restored to the normal position by approximately 10–11 weeks. Any abnormality after 11 weeks needs to be assessed carefully.

Exomphalos

The presence of a sac at the umbilicus with gut or liver contained in it is likely to be an exomphalos. The umbilical cord vessels can be seen traversing through this sac, which can vary in size. There is a strong association with chromosomal abnormality.

Bladder and cloacal extrophy

If the defect were to extend infraumbilically, it is likely to involve the fetal bladder (non-visualized bladder) and possibly the genitalia (ambiguous genitalia). Under these circumstances, post-natal surgery will involve extensive reconstruction of the urogenital system.

Beckwith–Wiedemann Syndrome

If the exomphalos is small with features of macrosomia and organomegaly in the fetus, a diagnosis of Beckwith–Wiedemann syndrome can be made and has implications for follow-up apart from surgery.

Pentalogy of Cantrell

If the anterior wall defect is more extensive superior to the umbilicus, it might involve parts of the diaphragm, pericardium, and the fetal heart as part of the Pentalogy of Cantrell.

Body-stalk anomaly

In some cases, a sac with the intra-abdominal contents is seen along with distortion of the spinal cord, poorly developed lower limbs, and a very short umbilical cord. These features form part of the body-stalk anomaly or amniotic rupture sequence and are uniformly associated with very poor prognosis.

Gastroschisis

The bowel is seen herniated without a sac (cauliflower-like appearance), just lateral to the cord insertion. Gastroschisis is usually located to the right of the umbilical cord, which has a normal insertion. The herniated organs usually only include loops of bowel and there is no association with chromosomal abnormality.

Bibliography

Barisic I, Clementi M, Hausler M, Gjergja R, Kern J, Stoll C, Euroscan Study Group. Evaluation of prenatal ultrasound diagnosis of fetal abdominal wall defects by 19 European registries. *Ultrasound Obstet Gynecol*. 2001; 18(4): 309–16.

Smrcek JM, Germer U, Krokowski M, Berg C, Krapp M, Geipel A, Gembruch U. Prenatal ultrasound diagnosis and management of body stalk anomaly: Analysis of nine singleton and two multiple pregnancies. *Ultrasound Obstet Gynecol*. 2003; 21(4): 322–8.

Williams DH, Gauthier DW, Maizels M. Prenatal diagnosis of Beckwith-Wiedemann syndrome. *Prenat Diagn*. 2005; 25(10): 879–84.

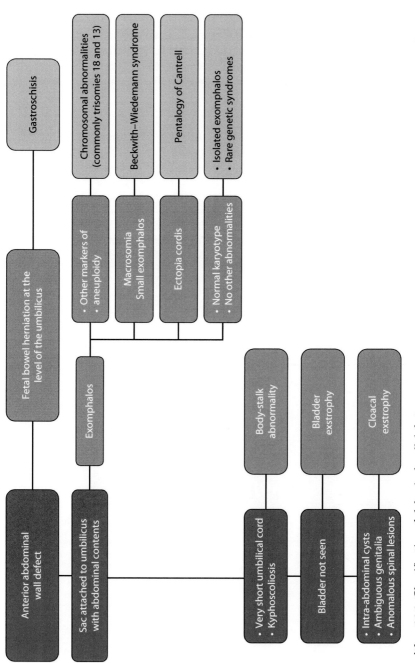

Algorithm 16.1 *Classification of abdominal wall defects.*

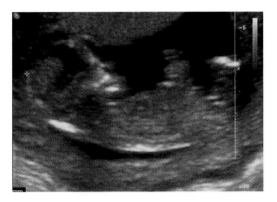

Figure 16.1 *First-trimester exomphalos.*

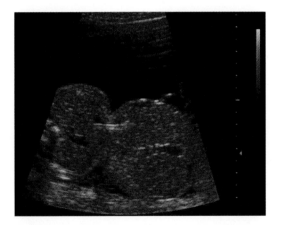

Figure 16.2 *Large exomphalos.*

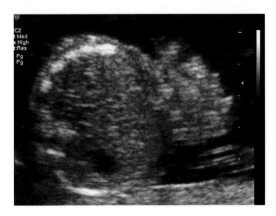

Figure 16.3 *Gastroschisis.*

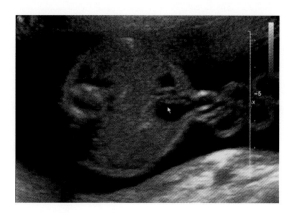

Figure 16.4 *Umbilical cord cyst.*

17

ABDOMINAL CYST

Cystic lesions in the fetal abdomen present either as isolated or multiple anechoic areas. The exact diagnosis of these is usually not possible antenatally. The outcome is dependent on the site and origin of these cysts and the presence of any associated abnormalities.

Isolated cystic lesions

Isolated cystic lesions are quite common and are usually considered benign. Their relationship to the fetal bladder usually gives a clue to their origin. Cystic lesion supero-lateral to the fetal bladder (frequently bilateral with septations) is suggestive of an ovarian cyst in a female fetus. In either sex, it could represent a mesenteric cyst or an intestinal duplication cyst. The occurrence of a cyst posterior to the bladder should raise the possibility of an anterior meningocele or hydrometrocolpos (female fetus). Rarely, the cyst may be seen totally unrelated to the bladder and in the upper abdomen. If these are in the right side, one should consider a benign liver cyst if the gallbladder is visualized and appears normal. The lack of an imageable gallbladder, especially on repeated scanning, suggests a choledochal cyst, which has more serious implications, such as associated biliary atresia.

Multiple lesions

Multiple lesions are usually either related to the fetal bowel or fetal kidneys (see Chapters 20 and 21). Typically, bowel obstruction manifests in the third trimester with multiple linear or discrete cystic spaces that connect with one another. Additionally, they have internal echoes that give a speckled appearance. Normal small intestine and colon measure approximately 7 and 20 mm in diameter, respectively. Any obvious dilatation beyond these limits needs to be followed up for evidence of bowel obstruction.

Duodenal atresia

A double bubble appearance in the fetal upper abdomen is suggestive of a high small intestinal obstruction most likely in the duodenum—duodenal atresia. This should prompt a thorough search for other markers as there is approximately a 1:3 risk for chromosomal abnormalities, and invasive prenatal diagnosis should be offered even if it is an isolated finding. Most other small intestinal obstructions are not related to chromosome abnormalities. They invariably tend to manifest in the third trimester and have progressive polyhydramnios needing drainage. The exact site(s) or cause (intrinsic, atresia, web, extrinsic [volvulus, peritoneal bands]) of obstruction(s) is not detectable ante-natally. Additional features such as echogenic bowel or ascitic fluid collection indicates meconium peritonitis and the prospective parents should be offered screening for cystic fibrosis.

Dilatation of the large bowel

Dilatation of the large bowel also manifests in the third trimester but is not usually associated with polyhydramnios. The suspicion of a large bowel obstruction such as anal atresia should prompt a thorough search for structural problems in all other systems as nearly 80% of these fetuses have associated anomalies.

First-trimester diagnosis

When diagnosed in the first trimester, detailed assessment of the fetal anatomy, including the heart, is necessary to rule out associated abnormalities. In cases with associated abnormalities, fetal karyotyping and echocardiography should be offered. If the cyst resolves, the parents can be reassured that the outcome is normal in the majority of cases. However, a post-natal assessment to exclude anorectal malformation should be arranged.

Bibliography

Hackmon-Ram R, Wiznitzer A, Gohar J et al. Prenatal diagnosis of a fetal abdominal cyst. *Eur J Obstet Gynecol Reprod Biol.* 2000; 91(1): 79–82.

Heling KS, Chaoui R, Kirchmair F et al. Fetal ovarian cysts: Prenatal diagnosis, management and postnatal outcome. *Ultrasound Obstet Gynecol.* 2002; 20(1): 47–50.

Khalil A, Cooke PC, Mantovani E et al. Outcome of first-trimester fetal abdominal cysts: Cohort study and review of the literature. *Ultrasound Obstet Gynecol.* 2014; 43: 413–9.

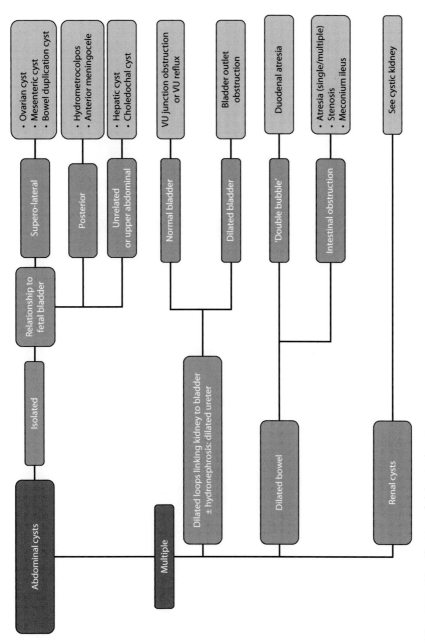

Algorithm 17.1 *Classification of abdominal cysts.*

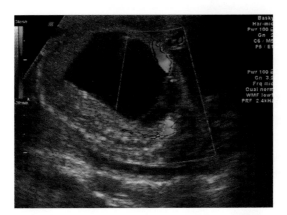

Figure 17.1 *Fetal ovarian cyst.*

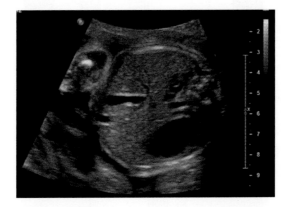

Figure 17.2 *Gallbladder.*

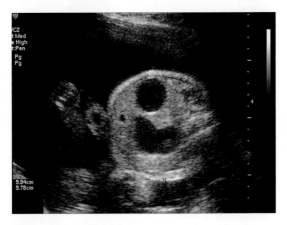

Figure 17.3 *Double bubble.*

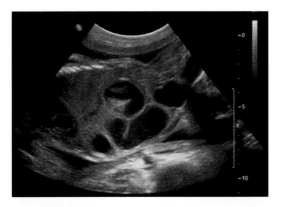

Figure 17.4 *Small bowel obstruction.*

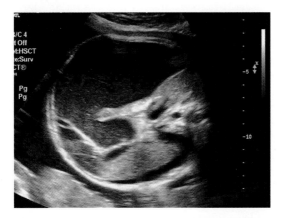

Figure 17.5 *Large bowel obstruction.*

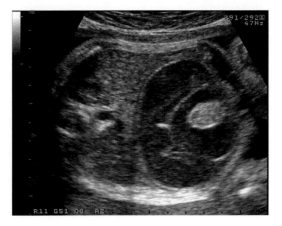

Figure 17.6 *Volvulus.*

18

ABDOMINAL ECHOGENICITY

The finding of increased echogenicity in the fetal abdomen is common. This may be in the fetal bowel, kidneys, or in the liver.

Echogenic bowel is the most common echogenic mass in the fetal abdomen. By definition the bowel is considered echogenic only if it is as bright as or brighter than the adjacent bone, namely, the iliac crest. The most common cause for echogenic bowel is fetal ingestion of blood cells. This is usually identified as floating particles in the amniotic fluid and is backed by history of vaginal bleeding. In the absence of any other markers for chromosomal markers or structural abnormalities, this isolated finding is unlikely to increase the risk for chromosomal abnormalities in a previously screened population, however, further screening options such as non-invasive prenatal tests and invasive diagnostic tests may be offered to the patient. The presence of associated bowel dilatation with or without ascitic fluid should raise the possibility of meconium peritonitis. This occurs when there is perforation of the bowel in utero and causes chemical peritonitis. This may be due to meconium ileus, and the couple should be offered screening for cystic fibrosis. Other causes are bowel atresia or volvulus, and these will be associated with bowel dilatation, which might manifest later on in the pregnancy.

Discrete isolated / single echogenic foci in the fetal abdomen are a relatively common finding at the routine anomaly scan. A thorough search should be made not only for other such foci in the brain, chest, etc., but also for any other markers for chromosomal or infective signs in the fetus. Typically, congenital infections such as varicella present with multiple foci in the liver and with additional features such as growth restriction, ventriculomegaly, etc. Screening for evidence of maternal infection can be considered for reassurance. If screening is negative, then a follow-up growth scan would identify any further developments such as an increase in the size of the foci, with significant vascularity suggesting a vascular malformation. This kind of change is extremely rare and is sporadically reported as hemangiomatous malformations in the liver, spleen, or rarely in the fetal adrenals. Usually, these foci manifest as isolated findings with no associated findings and have no impact on the outcome of the fetus.

Echogenic kidneys in the presence of dilated renal outflow tracts are suggestive of poor function in the kidneys. In the absence of any obvious outflow tract obstruction, the amniotic fluid volume should be assessed. If the fluid volume is indeed normal, then it is likely to be a physiological variant with a normal outcome. The presence of oligo or anhydramnios with bright kidneys suggests renal dysfunction and is likely to be associated with a poor outcome. Infantile polycystic kidneys usually manifest as large bright kidneys without any cortico-medullary differentiation. This invariably presents with anhydramnios and is a lethal malformation.

Bibliography

McNamara A, Levine D. Intra-abdominal fetal echogenic masses: A practical guide to diagnosis and management. *Radiographics*. 2005; 25(3): 633–45.

Sepulveda W, Leung KY, Robertson ME et al. Prevalence of cystic fibrosis mutations in pregnancies with fetal echogenic bowel. *Obstet Gynecol*. 1996; 87(1): 103–6.

Simchen MJ, Toi A, Bona M et al. Fetal hepatic calcifications: Prenatal diagnosis and outcome. *Am J Obstet Gynecol*. 2002; 187(6): 1617–22.

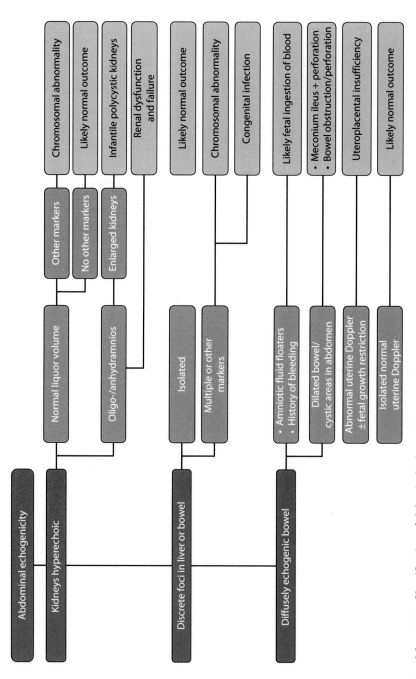

Algorithm 18.1 *Classification of abdominal echogenicity.*

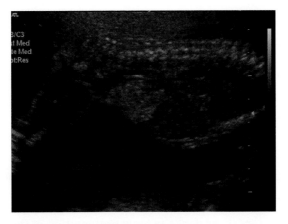

Figure 18.1 *Hyperechogenic bladder.*

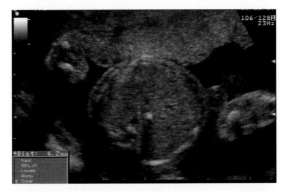

Figure 18.2 *Echogenic focus in liver.*

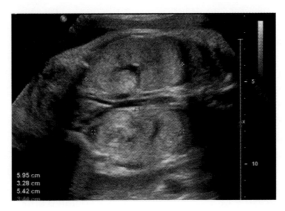

Figure 18.3 *Hyperechogenic kidneys.*

19

EMPTY RENAL FOSSA

The normal kidneys in fetal life are imaged in the renal fossae from about as early as 12 weeks of gestation.

Absence of renal tissue in the normal site, namely the renal fossa, may be due to true agenesis or due to ectopic presentation of the kidney. This could be either in the fetal pelvis or due to a fusion with the contralateral kidney. In either case, the kidney could show signs of pelvicalyceal dilatation due to the abnormal position and contour of the drainage system. In true agenesis, the renal artery is absent on the ipsilateral side. Ectopic kidneys derive their blood supply from the aorta or the iliac arteries. Unilateral agenesis is usually an isolated finding. However, it should prompt a thorough search for abnormalities in all organ systems. Presence of vertebral, limb, esophageal, or cardiac abnormalities would raise the suspicion of VATER or VACTERL associations. Presence of ambiguous genitalia or abnormal cystic lesions in the fetal pelvis could be MURCS association.

Bilateral renal agenesis is usually a diagnosis of exclusion, with the presentation being that of severe oligohydramnios or anhydramnios in the second trimester. The renal fossae are hard to image due to the lack of liquor. Additionally, the suprarenal glands occupy the renal fossae when the kidneys are not formed. These can mimic normal renal tissue on scan, thus making the diagnosis complicated. The lack of a normally filled bladder and renal arteries in the setting of anhydramnios would be features in favor of bilateral renal agenesis. The search for additional anomalies can be very challenging primarily due to the lack of liquor. In the majority of cases, the suspicion is usually only confirmed post-mortem, when associated abnormalities are also identified. The presence of cryptophthalmos and syndactyly would suggest the diagnosis of Fraser syndrome. Presence of vertebral, limb, esophageal, or cardiac abnormalities would raise the suspicion of VATER or VACTERL associations.

In general, unilateral agenesis of the kidney carries a good prognosis, provided the contralateral kidney appears to be structurally normal, with a normal bladder and liquor volume. In cases with bilateral agenesis, the outcome is uniformly fatal, regardless of the associated abnormalities. This is due to the lung hypoplasia as a consequence of the lack of amniotic fluid at the critical stage of lung development. In suspected bilateral agenesis, a post-mortem examination is invaluable in making a diagnosis and for predicting recurrence in future pregnancies.

Bibliography

Sepulveda W, Stagiannis KD, Flack NJ, Fisk NM. Accuracy of prenatal diagnosis of renal agenesis with color flow imaging in severe second-trimester oligohydramnios. *Am J Obstet Gynecol.* 1995; 173(6): 1788–92.

Yuksel A, Batukan C. Sonographic findings of fetuses with an empty renal fossa and normal amniotic fluid volume. *Fetal Diagn Ther.* 2004; 19(6): 525–32.

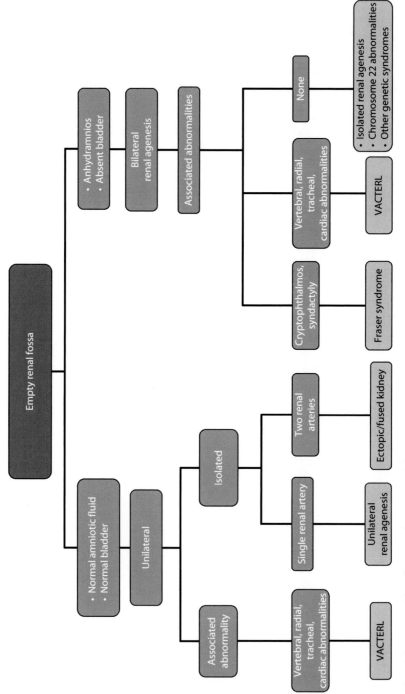

Algorithm 19.1 *Classification of empty renal fossa. VACTERL, vertebral, anal, cardiac, tracheo-esophageal, esophageal, renal, limb.*

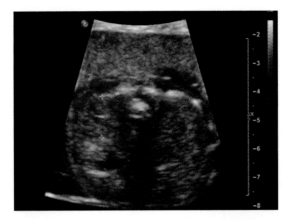

Figure 19.1 *Unilateral renal agenesis.*

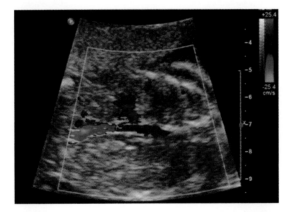

Figure 19.2 *Single renal artery in unilateral renal agenesis.*

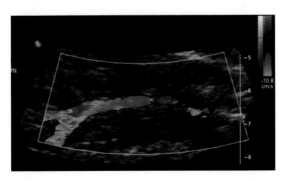

Figure 19.3 *Absent renal arteries in bilateral renal agenesis.*

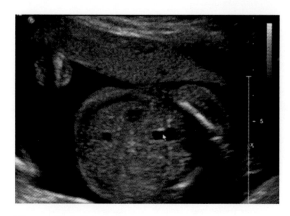

Figure 19.4 *Pelvic kidney.*

20

CYSTIC KIDNEY

Cystic kidney is a common finding in routine ante-natal screening. Presence of cysts in the renal cortex and increased echogenicity of the kidneys suggest the diagnosis of adult polycystic disease (autosomal dominant). In some, there might be demonstrable cysts in the fetal liver and spleen. The bladder and liquor volume are usually normal in this situation.

Multiple cysts with a dysplastic kidney could be in one or both kidneys. In this, there is no clear differentiation between cortex and medulla, the cysts are randomly distributed, and usually distort the renal outline. In general, unilateral multicystic kidney tends to be isolated and has a very good prognosis, provided the contralateral kidney is normal.

Bilateral multicystic kidneys are usually associated with anhydramnios or severe oligohydramnios, and this can compromise the assessment of the rest of the fetal anatomy due to poor visibility. Identification of macrosomia with a small exomphalos would suggest Beckwith-Wiedemann syndrome but is usually associated with normal or increased liquor. Multisystem abnormalities such as vertebral and cardiac abnormalities would suggest a diagnosis of VATER/VACTERL associations or chromosomal abnormalities such as trisomy 13 or 18. The presence of polydactyly along with an encephalocele would strongly suggest the possibility of Meckel–Gruber syndrome (autosomal recessive). A number of genetic syndromes are diagnosed after a post-natal assessment of the baby or after a post-mortem examination. Bilateral MCKD is a lethal condition, both because of the lack of normal renal function and pulmonary hypoplasia.

Absence of associated anomalies, normal chromosome study, and adequate amniotic fluid are all reassuring findings in cases of unilateral MCKD. A complete neonatal urologic work-up should be performed in all affected newborns.

Bibliography

Aubertin G, Cripps S, Coleman G et al. Prenatal diagnosis of apparently isolated unilateral multicystic kidney: Implications for counselling and management. *Prenat Diagn*. 2002; 22(5): 388–94.

van Eijk L, Cohen-Overbeek TE, den Hollander NS et al. Unilateral multicystic dysplastic kidney: A combined pre- and postnatal assessment. *Ultrasound Obstet Gynecol*. 2002; 19(2): 180–3.

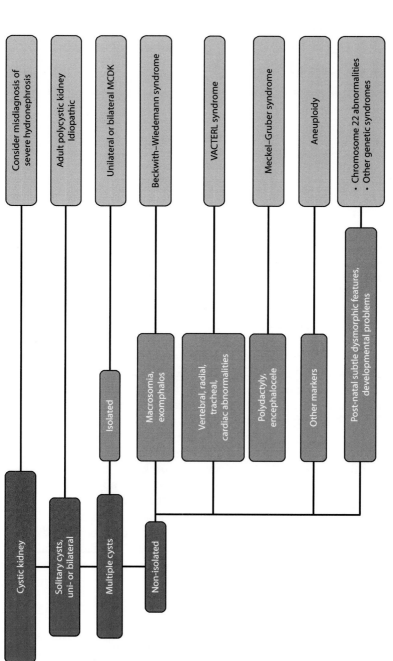

Algorithm 20.1 *Classification of cystic kidney. MCDK, multicystic dysplastic kidney; VACTERL, vertebral, anal, cardiac, tracheo-esophageal, esophageal, renal, limb.*

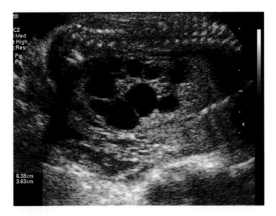

Figure 20.1 *Multicystic kidney.*

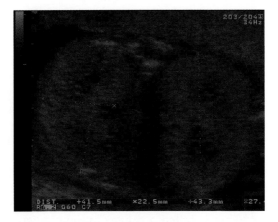

Figure 20.2 *Infantile polycystic kidney.*

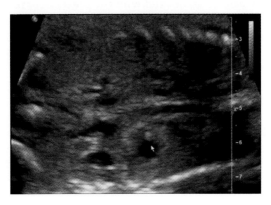

Figure 20.3 *Duplex kidney.*

21

FLUID-FILLED KIDNEY

Renal pelvis dilatation is present in approximately 1%–3% of all fetuses in mid-gestation. At the time of the 20 week routine anatomy scan it is defined as an A-P measurement of the renal pelvis of more than 4 mm or if there is calyceal dilatation.

The presence of hydronephrosis should prompt a thorough search for other soft markers for chromosomal abnormalities. In isolation, hydronephrosis does not increase the risk for chromosomal abnormalities. The entire urinary tract and amniotic fluid volume should also be assessed.

In the majority of cases (>85%), mild hydronephrosis is functional and resolves spontaneously during pregnancy or post-natally. In the remaining 15%, the condition is due to obstruction (usually at the pelvi-ureteric junction in unilateral hydronephrosis) or vesico-ureteric reflux. In this group there will usually be persistent hydronephrosis, and this measures >7 mm at >28 weeks with a proportion of babies needing post-natal corrective surgery. In all these cases, it is important to undertake post-natal assessment and imaging; these newborns also need prophylactic antibiotics until refluxing disease has been excluded.

Fluid in the kidney may sometimes be seen due to duplication of the collecting system. This is called a duplex system, where the kidney is drained by two ureters. When the cavities are not dilated it is a variant of normal, but it can also be associated with the presence of reflux (classically involving the lower pole ureter) or obstruction. A careful look for the presence of a ureterocele should also be undertaken.

In lower urinary tract obstruction, the hydronephrosis is accompanied by an enlarged bladder (megacystis), a dilated posterior urethra, and oligohydramnios after 16 weeks of gestation. The kidneys may appear dysplastic, with bright appearance and small cortical cysts. The finding has a high risk of perinatal mortality due to lethal pulmonary hypoplasia secondary to the absent amniotic fluid; there is a high chance of early-onset renal failure in the newborn. Fetal vesicoamniotic shunting may marginally improve perinatal survival but does not reduce the high rates of renal impairment in infancy, and longer term outcomes remain very poor.

Bibliography

Bhide A, Sairam S, Farrugia MK et al. The sensitivity of antenatal ultrasound for predicting renal tract surgery in early childhood. *Ultrasound Obstet Gynecol.* 2005; 25(5): 489–92.

Cheung KW, Morris RK, Kilby MD. Congenital urinary tract obstruction. *Best Pract Res Clin Obstet Gynaecol.* 2019 Jan 11. pii: S1521-6934(18)30202-5.

Sairam S, Al-Habib A, Sasson S et al. Natural history of fetal hydronephrosis diagnosed on mid-trimester ultrasound. *Ultrasound Obstet Gynecol.* 2001; 17(3): 191–6.

Whitten SM, McHoney M, Wilcox DT et al. Accuracy of antenatal fetal ultrasound in the diagnosis of duplex kidneys. *Ultrasound Obstet Gynecol.* 2003; 21(4): 342–6.

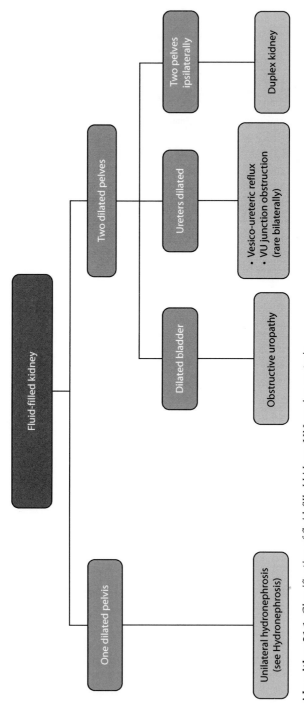

Algorithm 21.1 *Classification of fluid-filled kidney. VUJ, vesico-ureteric.*

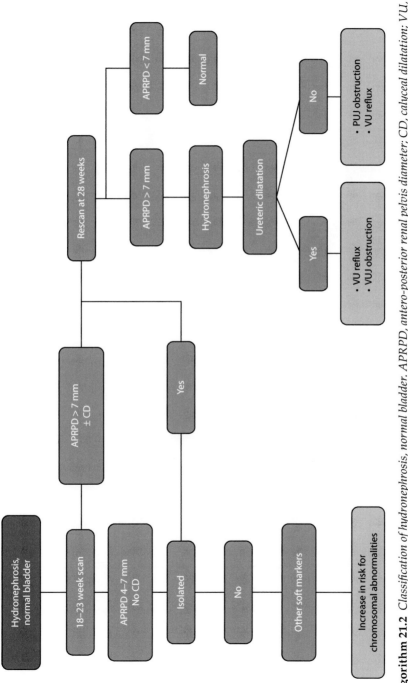

Algorithm 21.2 *Classification of hydronephrosis, normal bladder. APRPD, antero-posterior renal pelvis diameter; CD, calyceal dilatation; VU, vesico-ureteric; VUJ, vesico-ureteric junction; PUJ, pelvi-ureteric junction.*

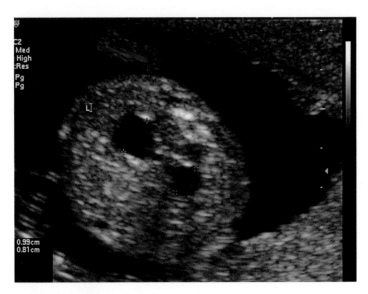

Figure 21.1 *Moderate hydronephrosis.*

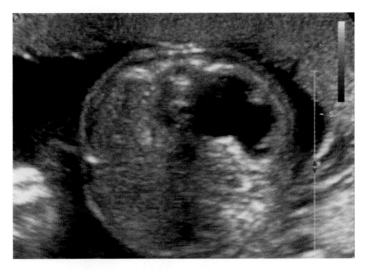

Figure 21.2 *Severe hydronephrosis.*

22

ECHOGENIC KIDNEYS

Kidneys are considered echogenic when they look brighter than the adjacent liver or spleen. The degree of echogenicity does not seem to be correlated with fetal outcome, and the difficulty is determining if the echogenic kidneys are a normal variant or an indicator of severe renal disease. The presence of positive family history of kidney disease is common in autosomal dominant polycystic kidney disease and, although typically the condition only manifests in adult life, early manifestation with pre-natal findings have been reported.

Non-isolated finding

In the presence of multiple fetal defects, an underlying chromosomal abnormality or genetic syndrome should be considered. Typical examples are Meckel–Gruber syndrome, VACTERL syndrome, and trisomy 13.

Abnormal amniotic fluid volume

The presence of oligo-anhydramnios, irrespective of the cause, dictates a poor prognosis. If the kidneys are enlarged and bright with oligohydramnios, the diagnosis of autosomal recessive polycystic kidney disease (ARPKD) should be considered. The prevalence is 1:30,000 and the risk of recurrence is 25%. Pre-natal diagnosis is available, but genetic testing of the index case is fundamental. The ultrasound diagnosis may not be possible before the late second or third trimester. If the kidneys are enlarged as well as the other measurements but the amniotic fluid remains normal, overgrowth syndromes like Beckwith–Wiedemann and Perlman syndromes should be considered.

Normal variants

Increased renal echogenicity with normal amniotic fluid and normal size kidneys is most likely a normal variant.

Bibliography

Mashiach R, Davidovits M, Eisenstein B et al. Fetal hyperechogenic kidney with normal amniotic fluid volume: A diagnostic dilemma. *Prenat Diagn*. 2005; 25(7): 553–58.

Winyard P, Chitty LS. Dysplastic and polycystic kidneys: Diagnosis, associations and management. *Prenat Diagn*. 2001; 21: 924–35.

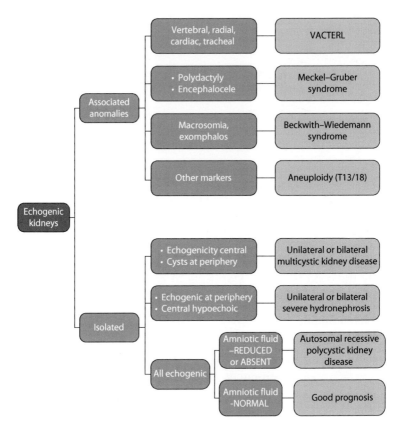

Algorithm 22.1 *Classification of echogenic kidneys.*

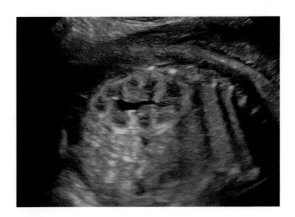

Figure 22.1 *Echogenic kidney.*

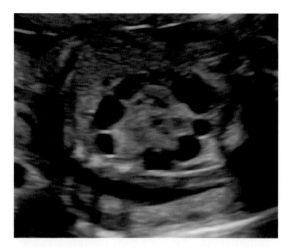

Figure 22.2 *Multicystic kidney.*

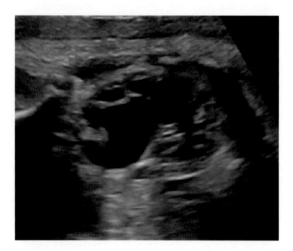

Figure 22.3 *Hydronephrosis.*

23

ENLARGED BLADDER

The fetal bladder can be easily visualized in all stages of pregnancy. Although the dimensions of the bladder are variable throughout the pregnancy, a longitudinal measurement of more than 7 mm in the first trimester is considered abnormal (megacystis). The bladder should always be assessed in combination with the liquor volume and the kidneys.

In the first trimester, megacystis should raise the suspicion of either chromosomal abnormalities or obstructive uropathy. Approximately 20% of fetuses with megacystis measuring between 7 and 15 mm have an underlying chromosomal abnormality such as trisomy 13 or 18. The majority of the fetuses with normal karyotype show spontaneous resolution of the bladder enlargement and have a normal outcome. If the bladder measures >15 mm, the risk of an underlying bladder outlet obstruction such as urethral atresia, posterior urethral valves, or cloacal abnormalities is very high and is associated with poor prognosis. In these fetuses it would be common to find abnormal kidneys (echogenic or dysplastic) along with significant reduction in the liquor volume even in the first trimester.

The finding of an enlarged bladder in the second trimester is usually due to bladder outlet obstruction. The presence of normal kidneys suggests that the renal function is likely to be preserved and is usually confirmed with the additional finding of normal liquor volume. These fetuses are likely to have intermittent outlet obstruction and tend to do well post-natally, provided the kidneys maintain their normal function throughout the pregnancy. With posterior urethral valves, there is usually incomplete or intermittent obstruction of the urethra, resulting in an enlarged and hypertrophied bladder with varying degrees of hydroureters, hydronephrosis, a spectrum of renal hypoplasia and dysplasia, oligohydramnios, and pulmonary hypoplasia. In some cases, there is associated urinary ascites from rupture of the bladder or transudation of urine into the peritoneal cavity.

The combination of an enlarged bladder with abnormal kidneys and reduced or absent liquor volume is indicative of poor renal function and is generally indicative of a guarded prognosis. The role of vesico-amniotic shunting remains controversial in these situations as the renal damage that is likely to have happened is irreversible.

Bibliography

Liao AW, Sebire NJ, Geerts L, Cicero S, Nicolaides KH. Megacystis at 10–14 weeks of gestation: Chromosomal defects and outcome according to bladder length. *Ultrasound Obstet Gynecol.* 2003; 21: 338–41.

Robyr R, Benachi A, Daikha-Dahmane F, Martinovich J, Dumez Y, Ville Y. Correlation between ultrasound and anatomical findings in fetuses with lower urinary tract obstruction in the first half of pregnancy. *Ultrasound Obstet Gynecol.* 2005; 25(5): 478–82.

Sepulveda W. Megacystis in the first trimester. *Prenat Diagn.* 2004; 24(2): 144–9.

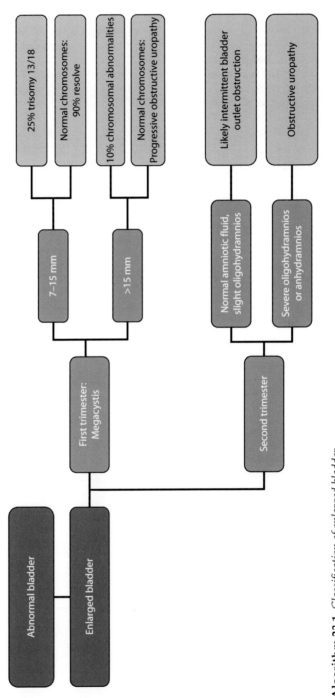

Algorithm 23.1 *Classification of enlarged bladder.*

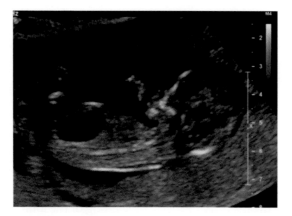

Figure 23.1 *Megacystitis.*

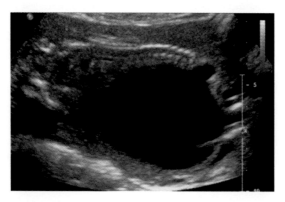

Figure 23.2 *Severe obstructive uropathy.*

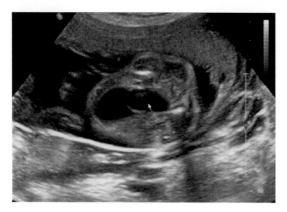

Figure 23.3 *Cystocele.*

24

SHORT LIMBS

Shortened femur length is the most common presentation for suspected skeletal problems as this is the only bone routinely measured in obstetric ultrasound. In the majority of cases, shortening of the long bones is likely to represent inaccurate dating, constitutional smallness, or an early feature of fetal growth restriction. The latter diagnosis must be excluded before contemplating a diagnosis of a fetal skeletal dysplasia—a heterogeneous group of disorders characterized by abnormalities of cartilage and bone growth. Typically, a diagnosis of a fetal skeletal dysplasia before 24 weeks results in a poor outcome due to thoracic dysplasia.

Fetal growth restriction

Approximately 10%–15% of short femur lengths noted at the 20–22 week anomaly scan will subsequently turn out to be due to severe early onset fetal growth restriction secondary to placental insufficiency. The finding of notched, high-resistance uterine artery Doppler is characteristic of this diagnosis.

Fetal aneuploidy

Short femur length is a marker for chromosomal abnormality. A thorough search for associated markers of aneuploidy should be undertaken.

Normal bone modeling (<24 weeks)

Unilateral femoral shortening is suggestive of focal femoral hypoplasia syndromes. Typically, the prognosis is good in most of these syndromes. The finding of bilateral shortening is suggestive of achondrogenesis. The latter is usually lethal associated with micromelia (extreme shortening of the entire limb) and thoracic dystrophy.

Abnormal bone modeling (<24 weeks)

Bowing may be difficult to differentiate from fractures of the long bones, but both suggest the diagnoses of achondrogenesis, thanatophoric dysplasia, campomelic dysplasia, or osteogenesis imperfecta. Definitive hypomineralization is indicative of either hypophosphatasia or osteogenesis imperfecta. Polydactyly is characteristic of short-ribbed polydactyly at this gestation and microcephaly occurs in chondrodysplasia punctata.

Third-trimester diagnosis

The most common diagnosis in the third trimester is achondroplasia. Spondyloepiphyseal dysplasias congenital (SEDC) is an alternative diagnosis, but this is rarely made pre-natally as the ultrasound features are subtle. The presence of polydactyly is suggestive of Jeune or Ellis–Van Creveld syndromes.

Bibliography

Lachman RS, Rappaport V. Fetal imaging in the skeletal dysplasias. *Clin Perinatol.* 1990; 17(3): 703–22.

Papageorghiou AT, Fratelli N, Leslie K, Bhide A, Thilaganathan B. Outcome of fetuses with antenatally diagnosed short femur. *Ultrasound Obstet Gynecol.* 2008; 31: 507–11.

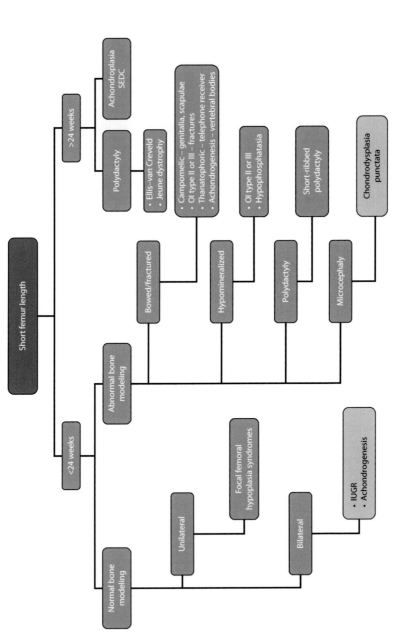

Algorithm 24.1 *Classification of short limbs. IUGR, intrauterine growth restriction; SEDC, spondyloepiphyseal dysplasia congenita; OI, osteogenesis imperfecta.*

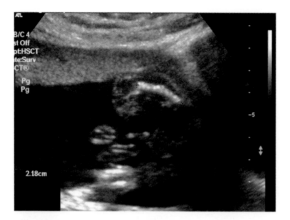

Figure 24.1 *Short bowed femur.*

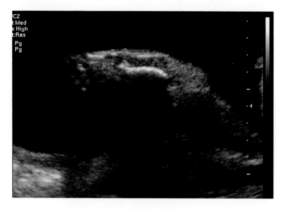

Figure 24.2 *Short bowed forearm.*

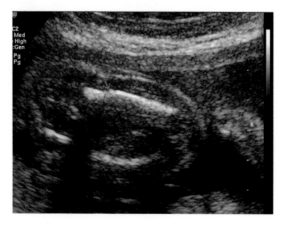

Figure 24.3 *Short fractured femur.*

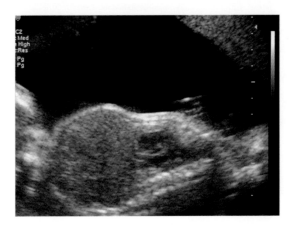

Figure 24.4 *Thoracic dystrophy.*

25

JOINT ABNORMALITIES

Typically, joint abnormalities are only diagnosed prenatally when they are severe. However, false positive diagnosis may be made due to natural joint mobility of fetuses and the effect of uterine crowding due to advanced pregnancy, oligohydramnios, or multiple pregnancy.

Talipes

Talipes is a varus deformity of the foot, which when diagnosed antenatally is due to abnormal innervation of the muscles of the ankle joint. When unilateral and isolated, the prognosis is very good. A significant proportion of complex/bilateral cases are associated with chromosomal abnormality, genetic syndromes, or neurodevelopmental disorders.

Fixed flexion of multiple joints

These findings fall under the umbrella term arthrogryposis multiplex congenital which covers many different neuromuscular disorders with guarded post-natal prognoses. The finding of cutaneous webs at the joints is typical of multiple pterygium syndrome. The confinement of abnormalities to the lower limb with an abrupt spinal termination is characteristic of caudal regression syndrome, often associated with diabetic pregnancy. If abnormalities in long bone length, mineralization, or fractures are seen, a skeletal dysplasia should be suspected.

Abnormal tone/posture

Rarely, abnormal posture or tone may be noted in the fetal joints suggesting a neuromuscular disorder, such as Pena–Shokeir sequence. The latter should only be suspected if the posture is persistently abnormal on several scans on different occasions.

Bibliography

Bakalis S, Sairam S, Homfray T, Harrington KF, Nicolaides K, Thilaganathan B. Outcome of antenatally diagnosed talipes equinovarus in an unselected obstetric population. *Ultrasound Obstet Gynecol* 2002; 20: 226–9.
Bonilla-Musoles F, Machado LE, Osborne NG. Multiple congenital contractures (congenital multiple arthrogryposis). *J Perinat Med*. 2002; 30(1): 99–104.

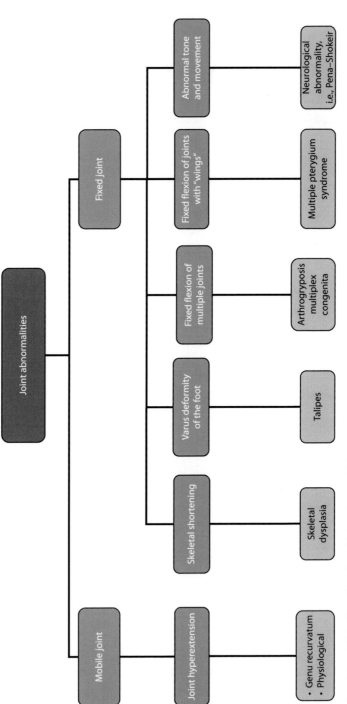

Algorithm 25.1 *Classification of joint abnormalities.*

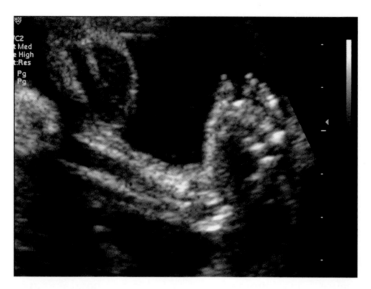

Figure 25.1 *Talipes.*

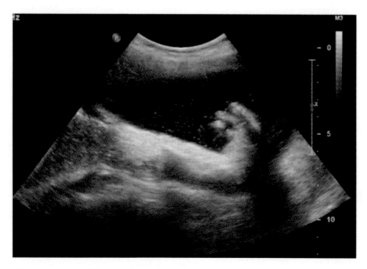

Figure 25.2 *Wrist contracture.*

26

HAND ABNORMALITIES

Typically, abnormalities of the hand are only noted as part of a careful fetal survey after the diagnosis of another abnormality. Under these circumstances, the hand abnormalities are likely to be related to the chromosomal or genetic abnormality diagnosed.

Abnormal hand movement/posture

The presence of overlapping fingers or a clenched hand is suggestive of a chromosomal disorder such as trisomy 18 or a neuromuscular disorder such as Pena–Shokeir sequence. If the hand is held in a decerebrate, inwardly turned posture, a radial array defect or neurodevelopmental problem should be suspected.

Abnormal hand structure

Polydactyly is a common isolated finding with an excellent prognosis. Associated features suggest a diagnosis such as a trisomy, skeletal dysplasia, Meckel–Gruber, and Smith–Lemli–Opitz syndromes. Missing or prematurely foreshortened digits are characteristic of amniotic band syndrome and terminal transverse limb defects. A split-hand or 'lobster-claw' deformity is suggestive of ectrodactyly.

Bibliography

Bromley B, Shipp TD, Benacerraf B. Isolated polydactyly: Prenatal diagnosis and perinatal outcome. *Prenat Diagn*. 2000; 20(11): 905–8.
Watson S. The principles of management of congenital anomalies of the upper limb. *Arch Dis Child*. 2000; 83(1): 10–7.

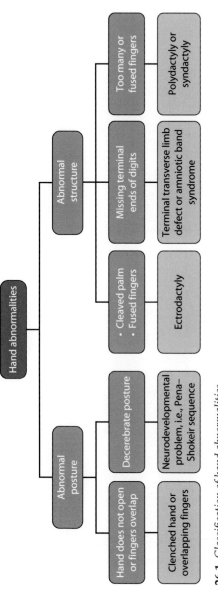

Algorithm 26.1 *Classification of hand abnormalities.*

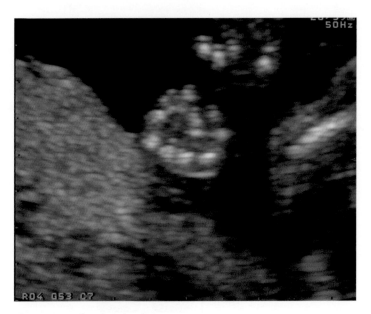

Figure 26.1 *Overlapping fingers.*

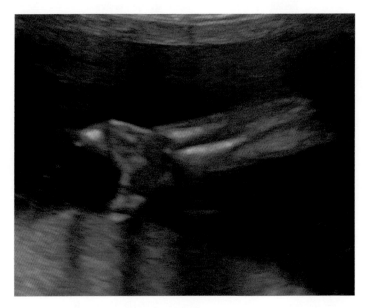

Figure 26.2 *Ectrodactyly of the hand.*

27

SPINAL ABNORMALITIES

The most common spinal abnormality encountered prenatally is spina bifida. Although other spinal lesions are possible, they are relatively infrequent.

Spina bifida

Typically, this is diagnosed on detection of the characteristic lemon-shaped head and "banana" cerebellum. The level of the lesion, the number of segments involved, severity of the kyphoscoliosis, ventriculomegaly, and microcephaly determine the prognosis for the neonate.

Sacrococcygeal teratoma

Sacrococcygeal teratoma usually presents as a vascular, semi-solid/semi-cystic tumor at the terminal end of the spine. Sacrococcygeal teratomas are associated with fetal hydrops and polyhydramnios from high-output cardiac failure related to the arterio-venous shunting within the tumor. These tumors are only rarely malignant, and the prognosis tends to be good after resection.

Spinal angulation

Hemivertebrae are rarely diagnosed prenatally probably because of the low prevalence and the relatively difficult ultrasound diagnosis. Most cases have a good prognosis, but consideration should be given to the diagnosis of VATER or VACTERL associations. Kyphosis (exaggerated hump) and scoliosis (lateral deformity) may be diagnosed prenatally as isolated abnormalities. Occasionally they may be associated with spina bifida, body stalk abnormality, and skeletal dysplasia.

Caudal regression

Caudal regression can vary in severity from partial sacral agenesis to complete absence of the lumbosacral spine. In an extreme form (sirenomelia), this presents with fusion and hypoplasia of the lower extremities and pelvic structures. Caudal regression occurs more commonly in diabetic pregnancy.

Bibliography

Mitchell LE, Adzick NS, Melchionne J et al. Spina bifida. *Lancet.* 2004 Nov 20–26; 364(9448): 1885–95.

Nyberg DA. The fetal central nervous system. *Semin Roentgenol.* 1990 Oct; 25(4): 317–33.

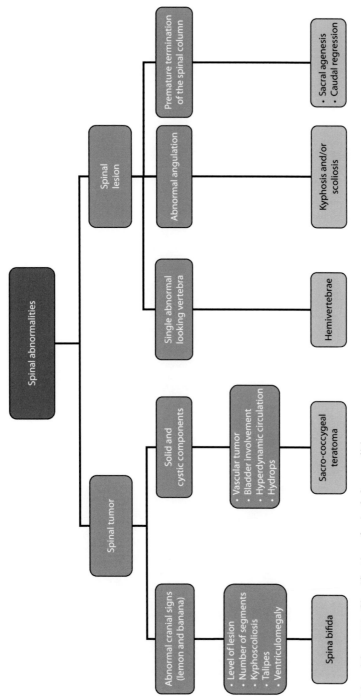

Algorithm 27.1 *Classification of spinal abnormalities.*

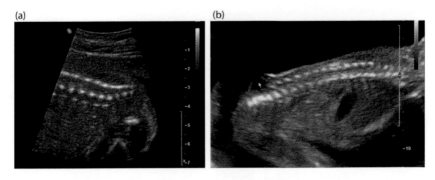

Figure 27.1 *(a) Normal spine. (b) Sacral meningomyelocele.*

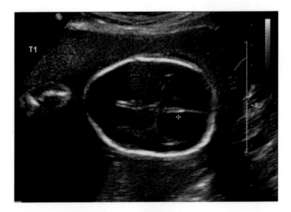

Figure 27.2 *Lemon-shaped head.*

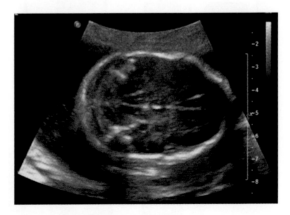

Figure 27.3 *"Banana" cerebellum.*

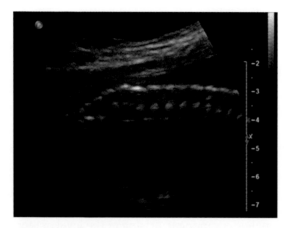

Figure 27.4 *Hemivertebrae.*

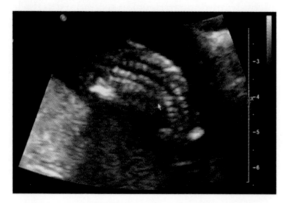

Figure 27.5 *Kyphoscoliosis.*

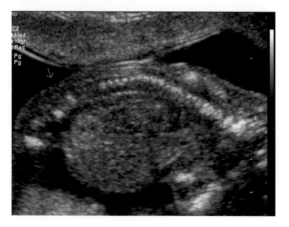

Figure 27.6 *Caudal regression.*

28

SPINAL MASSES

Sacrococcygeal teratomas are the most common fetal tumors with an incidence of about 1:40,000 births. These tumors are derived from multipotential embryonic cells, and most of them are external tumors with a variable pelvic component, arising at the level of sacrum at coccyx. They can be very large and are usually heterogenic with cystic and solid components. Polyhydramnios can develop secondary to the hyperdynamic circulation or in case of anemia secondary to intratumor bleeding. Most of the sacrococcygeal teratomas are benign with less than 10% showing a malignant component. Rapidly growing tumors, tumors with large intraperitoneal component, and the development of polyhydramnios or hydrops are associated with the worst prognosis.

Bibliography

Sananes N, Javadian P, Schwach Werneck Britto I et al. Technical aspects and effectiveness of percutaneous fetal therapies for large sacrococcygeal teratomas: Cohort study and literature review. *Ultrasound Obstet Gynecol*. 2016; 47: 712–9.

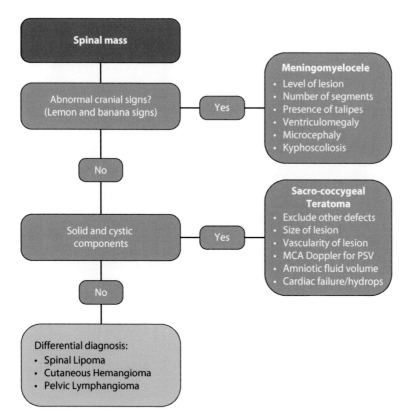

Algorithm 28.1 *Classification of spinal masses.*

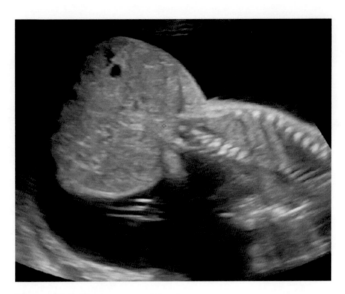

Figure 28.1 *Sacro-coccygeal teratoma.*

29

HEAD AND NECK MASSES

Fetal head and neck tumors are rare. When such masses are seen it is important to assess amniotic fluid volume, as polyhydramnios suggests problems with swallowing or obstruction. In addition, a careful survey of the fetal anatomy is necessary, as associated fetal abnormalities can suggest an underlying chromosomal or genetic syndrome.

The prognosis of these tumors largely depends on their size. If they are large, they can cause compression of the trachea, meaning that the airway in the newborn cannot be maintained. Careful monitoring of tumor size is necessary in order to decide whether ex utero intrapartum treatment (EXIT) needs to be performed at birth (see discussion later in this chapter). Other important factors for prognosis are the presence of associated abnormalities, fetal hydrops (possible in highly vascular tumors), and polyhydramnios (due to the risk of pre-term birth).

Cervical teratoma

This very rare tumor of the neck is made up of tissues that come from more than one embryonic layer (often including neural tissues, skin, cartilage, bone, and thyroid). This leads to a heterogeneous appearance on ultrasound. Usually tumors are unilateral, solid-cystic, multiloculated masses measuring 5–12 cm, with calcifications present in about half the cases. As they are large, they frequently cause airway obstruction, and this leads to polyhydramnios in 20%–40% of cases. Post-natal surgical correction usually involves extensive neck dissection, and frequently multiple procedures are necessary for complete resection and acceptable cosmetic results. In the long-term, infants are at risk of hypothyroidism and hypoparathyroidism.

Epignathus

This is a very rare oropharyngeal tumor classified as a mature teratoma. They arise from the sphenoid bone, palate pharynx, or jaw and grow into the oral and nasal cavities or into the cranium. On ultrasound there is a solid tumor in the oral cavity, and this is usually associated with polyhydramnios. The tumor is often very vascular, and this can lead to fetal cardiac decompensation and hydrops. The anatomy of the brain must be carefully examined as intracranial extension can occur. In addition, the tumor can be associated with cleft palate and micrognathia. The prognosis is poor due to airway obstruction, and the EXIT procedure is usually required.

Fetal goiter

This is an enlargement of the fetal thyroid gland. It can be due to maternal hyperthyroidism or hypothyroidism, but has also been reported in euthyroid women. Ultrasound features are of a symmetrical anterior solid mass, which can result in hyperextension of the fetal head. The goiter can cause polyhydramnios, and hyperextension can lead to dystocia. In most cases there is a history of maternal thyroid disease, and maternal therapy will usually cause improvement in fetal hyperthyroidism. In some cases, fetal blood sampling may be necessary to determine the fetal thyroid status, and direct fetal therapy by amniocentesis or cordocentesis has been reported.

Cystic hygroma

This is the most common cause for an ante-natal finding of a neck mass and is thought to be due to lymphatic malformation. In the first trimester, cystic hygromas can be identified as increased nuchal translucency at the 11–13^{+6} week scan (see Chapter 30). Second-trimester diagnosis is by an ultrasound finding of a thin-walled cystic swelling at the back of the neck with a characteristic midline septum (the nuchal ligament). Often there are multiple septa, and the swelling is frequently symmetrical. Cystic hygromas can become very large and, in these cases, can extend anteriorly, into the axilla or mediastinum. The presence of hydrops fetalis is a poor prognostic indicator, associated with a mortality rate >95%. Fetal cystic hygromas are strongly associated with underlying chromosomal abnormalities (in particular Turner syndrome and fetal trisomy) and genetic syndromes (e.g., Noonan syndrome, Joubert syndrome). Detailed ultrasound examination including fetal echocardiography for other features of these abnormalities should be performed, and the parents should be offered the option of fetal karyotyping. Hygromas that are small and those discovered late in pregnancy have a better prognosis. Of these, many resolve spontaneously, and post-natal treatment is to improve mechanical obstruction and cosmesis.

Fetal hemangioma

Fetal hemangioma affecting the neck or face is a rare condition and appears on ultrasound as a thick-walled sonolucent mass in which characteristic pulsating Doppler flow signals are detected. At birth, there is a purplish tumor with ectatic vessels. Classically this is fully developed at birth and rapidly regresses within 6–18 months.

Ex Utero Intrapartum Treatment (EXIT)

This procedure is used in fetuses with large neck masses or laryngotracheal atresia, due to the high mortality associated with a delay in obtaining an airway and achieving effective ventilation. The aim of the procedure is to allow time to secure the airway of the newborn while maintaining utero-placental gas exchange. This is achieved by endotracheal intubation or tracheostomy, although bronchoscopy and resection of the neck mass have been described.

In cases of polyhydramnios, amnioreduction before the procedure has been described to prevent decompression and contraction of the uterus. General anesthesia with pharmacological uterine relaxation in order to preserve placental function is achieved prior to Caesarean section. Careful hemostasis is ensured during the procedure, and the uterus is opened using a uterine stapling device in order to minimize blood loss. The fetus is delivered while the intact utero-placental circulation continues to provide gas exchange, and the airway is secured prior to clamping of the cord.

Bibliography

Gallagher PG, Mahoney MJ, Gosche JR. Cystic hygroma in the fetus and newborn. *Semin Perinatol.* 1999 Aug; 23(4): 341–56.

Noah MM, Norton ME, Sandberg P, Esakoff T, Farrell J, Albanese CT: Short-term maternal outcomes that are associated with the EXIT procedure, as compared with cesarean delivery. *Am J Obstet Gynecol.* 2002; 186(4): 773–7.

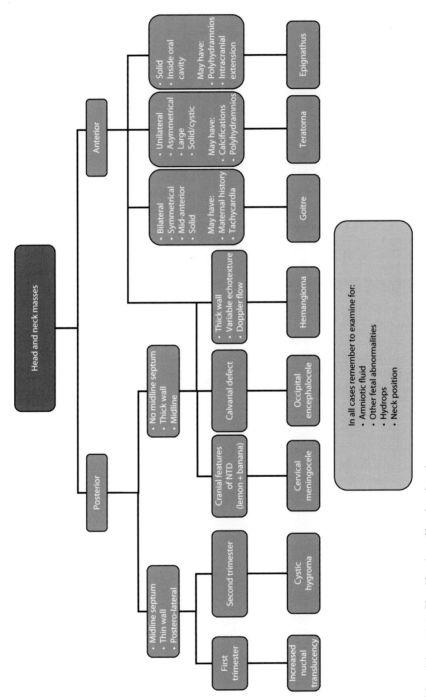

Algorithm 29.1 *Classification of head and neck masses.*

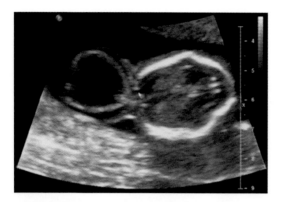

Figure 29.1 *Encephalocele.*

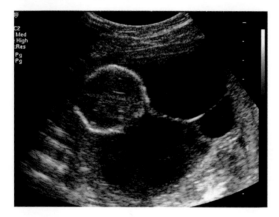

Figure 29.2 *Cystic hygroma.*

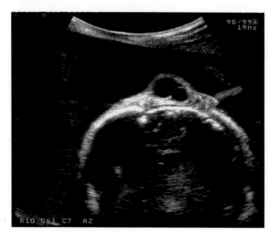

Figure 29.3 *Facial cyst.*

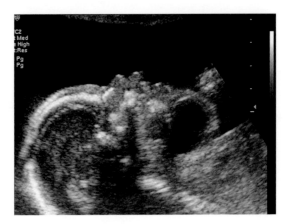

Figure 29.4 *Neck tumor.*

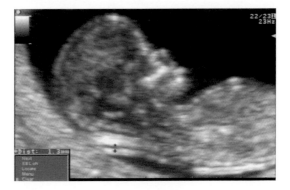

Figure 29.5 *Normal nuchal measurement.*

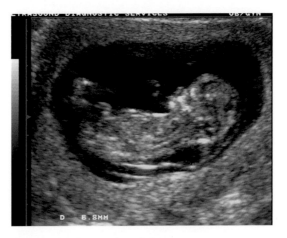

Figure 29.6 *Increased nuchal measurement.*

30

INCREASED NUCHAL TRANSLUCENCY

All fetuses have a collection of fluid under the skin behind the neck at $11-13^{+6}$ weeks of gestation. This nuchal translucency (NT) is visible and measurable on ultrasound. There are many causes for increased NT, and there may not be a single underlying mechanism for its presence.

Chromosomal abnormalities

Nuchal translucency (NT) is the single most important marker for chromosomal abnormalities in the first trimester and by far the most widely researched. Screening for trisomy 21 by combining NT with maternal age and maternal serum biochemistry results in a detection rate of about 80% of cases for a 3% invasive testing rate. The NT is increased in other chromosomal abnormalities, and a screening program for trisomy 21 will also detect the majority of fetuses with other trisomies.

Cardiac defects

Heart abnormalities are associated with increased NT thickness in chromosomally normal fetuses. The prevalence of heart abnormalities is about 7% if the NT is 4.5–5.4 mm, 20% for NT of 5.5–6.4 mm, and 30% for NT of 6.5 mm or more. Using NT as a screening test for major heart defects will significantly improve detection rates for cardiac abnormalities. In pregnancies with increased NT, specialist fetal echocardiography should be considered for fetuses with an NT higher than the 95th percentile.

Fetal abnormalities and movement disorders

Increased fetal NT is associated with a high prevalence of major fetal abnormalities. There is a long and growing list of abnormalities associated with increased NT, and common defects include hydrops, congenital diaphragmatic hernia, exomphalos, body stalk anomaly, skeletal abnormalities, and fetal movement disorders such as fetal akinesia deformation sequence. A careful anatomical survey should therefore be performed in chromosomally normal fetuses with increased NT.

Genetic syndromes

Increased NT has been associated with a large number of genetic syndromes. The rarity of these means that it can be difficult to establish whether the observed prevalence is higher than the general population, but it appears that congenital adrenal hyperplasia, fetal akinesia deformation sequence, Noonan syndrome, Smith–Lemli–Opitz syndrome, and spinal muscular atrophy are more prevalent than expected in the general population.

Bibliography

Makrydimas G, Sotiriadis A, Huggon IC et al. Nuchal translucency and fetal cardiac defects: A pooled analysis of major fetal echocardiography centers. *Am J Obstet Gynecol.* 2005 Jan; 192(1): 89–95.
Snijders RJ, Noble P, Sebire N et al. UK multicentre project on assessment of risk of trisomy 21 by maternal age and fetal nuchal-translucency thickness at 10–14 weeks of gestation. Fetal Medicine Foundation First Trimester Screening Group. *Lancet.* 1998 Aug 1; 352(9125): 343–6.

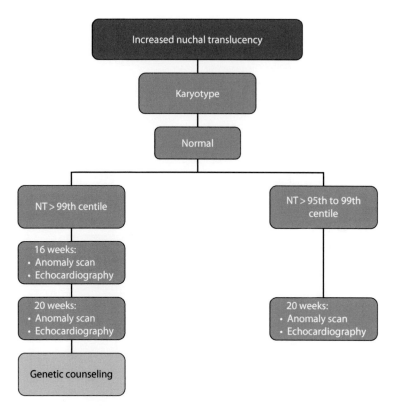

Algorithm 30.1 *Classification of increased nuchal translucency.*

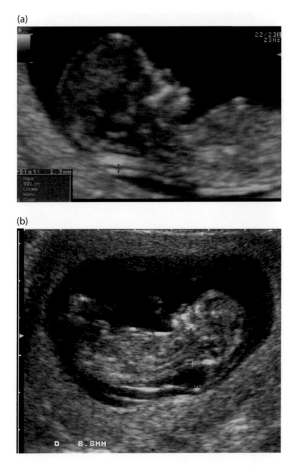

Figure 30.1 *(a) Normal nuchal measurement. (b) Increased nuchal measurement.*

31

PLACENTAL ABNORMALITIES

Molar pregnancy

Hydatidiform mole can be categorized as complete (where there is absence of a fetus) and incomplete (where a fetus is present). The majority of molar pregnancies miscarry spontaneously in the first trimester, and only rarely will cases reach the second trimester. Complete moles result from fertilization of an empty ovum by sperm which then duplicates its chromosomes. In some cases, the enucleated egg is fertilized by two sperms (dispermy). In incomplete or partial mole, fertilization of a normal ovum occurs and there is duplication of the paternal chromosomes, or from dispermy, resulting in triploidy. Ultrasound shows the placenta to be an enlarged complex intrauterine mass containing many small cysts which can be described as grape-like (hydatidiform).

Placental lakes

Placental lakes appear as sonolucent areas in the placenta. They are often associated with fetal growth restriction due to placental insufficiency. However, they are commonly seen in normal pregnancy and are more common with advancing gestation and increasing placental thickness. Prospective studies examining the outcomes of pregnancies with placental lakes have failed to show a consistent association with utero-placental complications or adverse pregnancy outcome.

Jelly-like placenta

Rarely, the placenta can appear thick, with a patchy echogenicity. "Jelly-like" refers to the placenta quivering like jelly to sharp abdominal pressure. The finding has been reported as being strongly associated with adverse pregnancy outcome. Therefore, it may be advisable to perform serial growth scans in such cases.

Grading

Grannum et al. proposed a method of grading of placental appearance in 1979. The original classification of placental maturity was correlated to fetal lung maturity as assessed by the lecithin-sphingomyelin (L/S) ratio. Subsequent studies reported that in pregnancies complicated with intrauterine growth retardation, there is premature appearance of grade III placenta, and that this premature appearance is more common in smokers and the young. While there is some correlation between placental and lung maturity, placental grading is limited by the wide variation in the progression of placental maturation. Placental grading was used in order to identify pregnancies at risk before the wide availability of Doppler equipment. This shift to the use of Doppler, the poor inter-observer agreement for placental grading, and the poor correlation of placental grade to neonatal outcome has meant that the effectiveness of reporting Grannum grades in clinical practice is limited and largely historical.

Chorioangioma

Although chorioangioma is the most common tumor of the placenta, it is rare—occurring in about 1:5,000–10,000 pregnancies. It is a vascular malformation, usually seen as a circumscribed solid mass that may protrude from the fetal surface of the placenta. Intraplacental tumors are more difficult to recognize, and targeted ultrasound using color Doppler can help in identifying chorioangiomas in cases with a high index of suspicion, for example in unexplained polyhydramnios or hydrops with evidence of hyperdynamic fetal blood flow. Pregnancies complicated by placental chorioangioma are at increased risk of polyhydramnios and associated pre-term delivery. In more severe cases, fetal hydrops can occur, and Doppler investigation of the middle cerebral artery can show high peak velocity blood flow indistinguishable from fetal anemia. Such pregnancies are at high risk of fetal demise, and treatment with amniodrainage in order to prevent pre-term delivery or interstitial laser ablation may be successful in improving perinatal outcome. Apart from the effects of a hyperdynamic circulation, associations with chorioangioma include fetal growth restriction, placental abruption, and umbilical artery thrombosis.

Bibliography

Reis NS, Brizot ML, Schultz R et al. Placental lakes on sonographic examination: Correlation with obstetric outcome and pathologic findings. *J Clin Ultrasound*. 2005 Feb; 33(2): 67–71.

Sau A, Seed P, Langford K. Intraobserver and interobserver variation in the sonographic grading of placental maturity. *Ultrasound in Obstetrics and Gynecology*. 2004; 23(4): 374–7.

Sepulveda W, Alcalde JL, Schnapp C et al. Perinatal outcome after prenatal diagnosis of placental chorioangioma. *Obstet Gynecol*. 2003 Nov; 102(5 Pt 1): 1028–33.

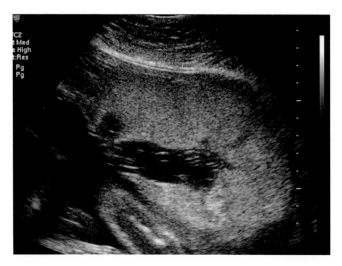

Figure 31.1 *Placental lakes.*

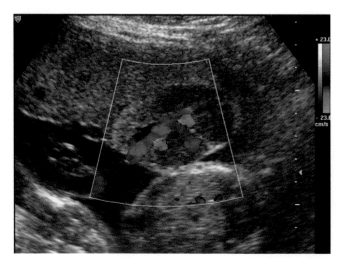

Figure 31.2 *Placental chorioangioma.*

32

SINGLE UMBILICAL ARTERY

The normal umbilical cord contains two arteries and one vein. A single umbilical artery (SUA) occurs in around 1% of cords in singletons. Ante-natal diagnosis can be by examination of a transverse section of the cord using B-mode or by using color flow Doppler imaging of the superior vesical arteries (intra-abdominal origin of the umbilical arteries), which are normally visualized on each side of the fetal bladder.

Consequences

About 20%–30% of fetuses with a single umbilical artery have associated abnormalities. The commonly reported defects are cardiovascular abnormalities (especially ventricular septal defects and cono-truncal defects), abdominal wall defects, and urinary tract abnormalities. In addition, there is a higher incidence of marginal and velamentous insertion of the umbilical cord. There is also an increased risk of intrauterine or neonatal death, but most of these deaths occur in those with associated congenital abnormalities. Most (but not all) studies report higher risks—less so in apparently isolated single umbilical artery cases. Adverse outcomes relate to intrauterine growth restriction (IUGR) and pre-term birth, leading to a perinatal mortality rate which is 5–10 times higher. Reference ranges for umbilical artery Doppler do not apply to cases with a single umbilical artery, where the resistance is typically lower. Elevated umbilical artery pulsatility index (PI) in cases of a single umbilical artery is obviously abnormal, but a normal PI is not reassuring.

Chromosomal abnormalities

A single umbilical artery is more commonly seen in trisomy 18, trisomy 13, and triploidy. These are almost always associated with multiple abnormalities, and in a low-risk patient the finding of an isolated single umbilical artery does not significantly increase the risk for a chromosomal defect.

Management

Prenatal diagnosis of a single umbilical artery should prompt careful examination for other abnormalities, and, in particular, fetal echocardiography should be performed, as heart defects are more common. Fetal karyotyping should be considered depending on the presence of fetal abnormalities and prior risk. Serial ultrasound examination to ensure linear fetal growth should be performed in ongoing cases. The pediatric team should be made aware prior to routine post-natal examination, as there is an increased proportion of significant occult renal malformations in asymptomatic infants born with apparently isolated SUA, with a significant proportion affected with vesico-ureteric reflux.

Bibliography

Predanic M, Perni SC, Friedman A et al. Fetal growth assessment and neonatal birth weight in fetuses with an isolated single umbilical artery. *Obstet Gynecol.* 2005 May; 105(5 Pt 1): 1093–7.

Srinivasan R, Arora RS. Do well infants born with an isolated single umbilical artery need investigation? *Arch Dis Child.* 2005 Jan; 90(1): 100–1.

Thummala MR, Raju TN, Langenberg P. Isolated single umbilical artery anomaly and the risk for congenital malformations: A meta analysis. *J Pediatr Surg.* 1998; 33(4): 580–585.

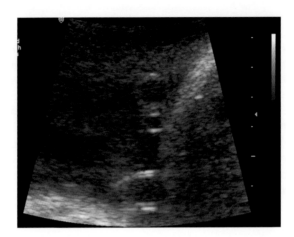

Figure 32.1 *Single umbilical artery.*

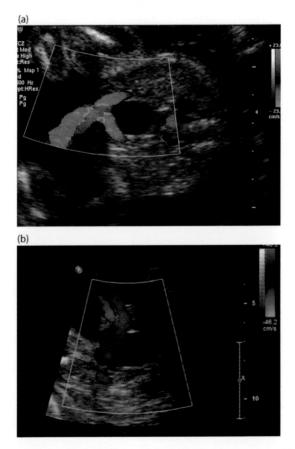

Figure 32.2 *(a) Two umbilical arteries on color Doppler. (b) Single umbilical artery on color Doppler.*

33

OLIGOHYDRAMNIOS AND ANHYDRAMNIOS

Oligohydramnios occurs in 0.5%–1% of pregnancies. The diagnosis is usually made subjectively. It is defined as an amniotic fluid index (AFI) of less than 5 cm or a deepest single pocket measurement of 1 cm or less. Anhydramnios means that no amniotic fluid is seen.

Amniotic fluid is mainly produced by fetal urine. Before 16 weeks the placenta contributes significantly and therefore oligohydramnios is unusual before mid-gestation, with the exception of rupture of membranes (ROM). Oligohydramnios is caused because there is reduced production of fetal urine (e.g., placental insufficiency, renal agenesis), because the fetus cannot urinate due to obstruction (e.g., posterior urethral valves), or because the fluid that is produced drains away due to rupture of membranes (ROM). As with all abnormalities, targeted detailed ultrasound for associated abnormalities should be performed. The prognosis depends on the cause. The absence of fluid and associated abnormal posturing of the fetus can make examination for fetal abnormalities difficult.

A lack of amniotic fluid can lead to pulmonary hypoplasia due to compression of the chest and abdomen and limitation of movement of the diaphragm, and after birth this leads to death from severe respiratory insufficiency. Marked fetal deformation due to fetal compression including a flattened face, hypertelorism, low-set ears, and micrognathia (Potter syndrome) can occur in renal agenesis and multicystic/polycystic kidneys as well as some obstructive uropathies. Rupture of membranes at less than 20 weeks is associated with a very poor outcome due to a high chance of pulmonary hypoplasia. These pregnancies carry the additional risks of miscarriage/pre-term birth and ascending infection, and overall survival is less than 10%. Fetal growth restriction due to placental insufficiency which presents at 20–24 weeks is likely to be severe, with a high risk in perinatal mortality.

Treatment of pre-term ROM at less than 26 weeks of gestation with serial amnioinfusion has been reported as improving the outcome in some cases, but this requires further evaluation. Pre-natal treatment of obstructive uropathy with vesico-ureteric shunting has been reported. This was reported to lead to an improved survival but also a high chance of end-stage renal disease in neonatal periods and early childhood. A randomized controlled trial reported that the chance of newborn babies surviving with normal renal function is very low irrespective of whether vesico-amniotic shunting is done. Therefore, caution should be exercised with pre-natal intervention.

Bibliography

Biggio JR Jr, Wenstrom KD, Dubard MB, Cliver SP. Hydramnios prediction of adverse perinatal outcome. *Obstet Gynecol.* 1999; 94: 773–7.

Locatelli A, Vergani P, Di Pirro G, Doria V, Biffi A, Ghidini A. Role of amnioinfusion in the management of premature rupture of the membranes at <26 weeks' gestation. *Am J Obstet Gynecol.* 2000; 183: 878–82.

Morris RK, Malin GL, Quinlan-Jones E et al. Percutaneous vesicoamniotic shunting in Lower Urinary Tract Obstruction (PLUTO) Collaborative Group. Percutaneous vesicoamniotic shunting versus conservative management for fetal lower urinary tract obstruction (PLUTO): A randomised trial. *Lancet.* 2013; 382(9903): 1496–506.

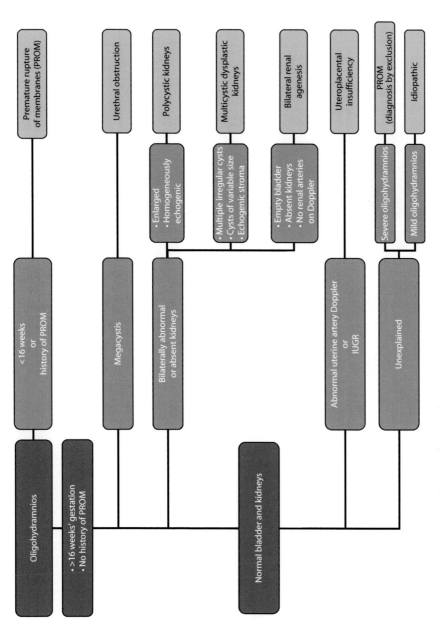

Algorithm 33.1 *Classification of oligohydramnios.*

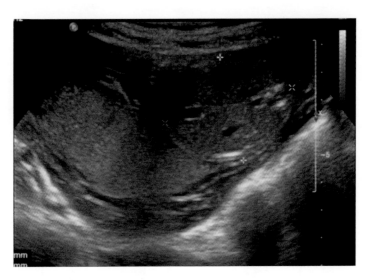

Figure 33.1 *Anhydramnios.*

34

POLYHYDRAMNIOS

Polyhydramnios is caused by reduced fetal swallowing or increased fetal urine production. This occurs in 0.5%–1% of pregnancies. The diagnosis is usually made subjectively. It is defined as an amniotic fluid index (AFI) of more than 24 cm or a deepest single pocket measurement of fluid of at least 8 cm. The prognosis depends on the cause, but the perinatal mortality rate is about two to three times that of pregnancies with normal amniotic fluid volume even in the absence of fetal defects. If polyhydramnios is associated with a fetal or placental malformation, the perinatal mortality is as high as 60%.

Complications include pre-term labor, which affects up to one in four cases, malpresentation and need for Caesarean section, placental abruption, and post-partum hemorrhage. Amniodrainage for polyhydramnios is aimed at reducing the risk of pre-term delivery and improving maternal discomfort. As with all defects, targeted detailed ultrasound for associated abnormalities should be performed. There are associated fetal abnormalities in about 20% of cases.

Fetal structural abnormalities

The most common associated defects are gastrointestinal or central nervous system abnormalities. The presence of multiple abnormalities or abnormalities that do not explain the polyhydramnios should raise the suspicion of an underlying chromosomal or genetic syndrome. In cases of obstruction, such as gastrointestinal or pulmonary abnormalities, polyhydramnios can be very severe and recur quickly after amniodrainage, often necessitating serial drainages.

Fetal movement disorders

Absent or greatly reduced fetal movement can be suggestive of a (typically progressive) neuromuscular disorder.

Placental tumors

The presence of a placental tumor, such as a chorioangioma, may cause a hyperdynamic circulation, which leads to a high peak systolic velocity (PSV) in the middle cerebral artery (MCA).

Fetal anemia

Doppler examination of the MCA reveals a high PSV. Fetal edema, ascites, or hydrops may be present if the anemia is severe. The mother may have a history of alloimmune antibodies or there may be a history or blood results suggestive of parvovirus infection. Fetal anemia can be treated by fetal blood transfusion. In immune mediated anemias, repeat transfusions will usually be required, while in parvovirus, a single transfusion is usually sufficient due to fetal recovery from the disease.

Arrhythmias

Careful examination of the fetal heart including the heart rhythm should be performed in order to exclude conditions such as fetal supraventricular tachycardia or heart block. Treatment is indicated if there are signs of fetal compromise, such as hydrops fetalis. Many fetal arrhythmias can be treated by maternal administration of an anti-arrhythmic drug (transplacental treatment).

Bibliography

Biggio JR Jr, Wenstrom KD, Dubard MB et al. Hydramnios prediction of adverse perinatal outcome. *Obstet Gynecol.* 1999 Nov; 94(5 Pt 1): 773–7.
Locatelli A, Vergani P, Di Pirro G et al. Role of amnioinfusion in the management of premature rupture of the membranes at <26 weeks' gestation. *Am J Obstet Gynecol.* 2000 Oct; 183(4): 878–82.
Newbould MJ, Lendon M, Barson AJ. Oligohydramnios sequence: The spectrum of renal malformations. *Br J Obstet Gynaecol.* 1994 Jul; 101(7): 598–604.

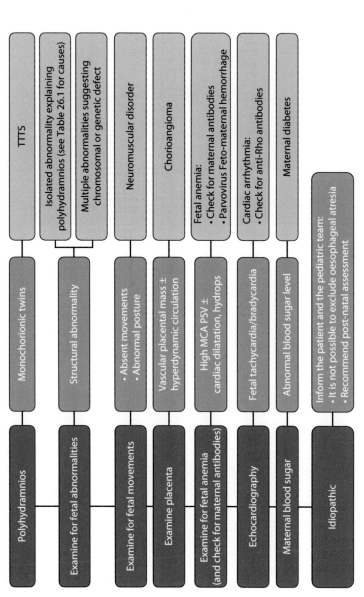

Algorithm 34.1 *Classification of polyhydramnios. MCA PSV, middle cerebral artery peak systolic velocity; TTTS, twin–twin transfusion syndrome.*

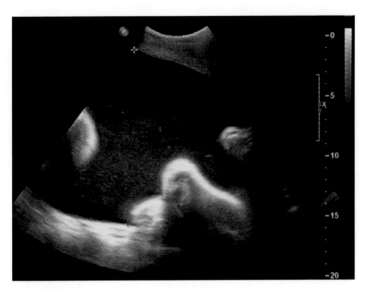

Figure 34.1 *Polyhydramnios.*

35

AMNIOTIC BANDS

Amniotic bands occur as a consequence of a disruption to the amnion with an intact chorion. In most cases, amniotic bands occur without any associated fetal effects, though occasionally a diagnosis of amniotic band syndrome may be made because of associated fetal anomalies. Amniotic band syndrome is believed to be caused by entrapment of fetal parts (usually a limb or digits) in fibrous amniotic membrane while in utero. When the amnion ruptures, fetal parts may protrude into the extra-embryonic coelom and the amniotic membrane can entangle various fetal parts, thereby reducing blood supply and causing congenital abnormalities (typically resulting in amputations). Although no two cases are exactly alike, there are several features that are relatively common: syndactyly, distal ring constrictions, shortened bone growth, limb length discrepancy, distal lymphedema, and congenital bands. Very confusingly, by the time amniotic band syndrome is suspected, the amniotic bands are no longer visible, as the fetal insult probably occurred early in the first trimester.

Bibliography

Lockwood C, Ghidini A, Romero R et al. Amniotic band syndrome: Re-evaluation of its pathogenesis. *Am J Obstet Gynecol* 1989; 160: 1030–3.

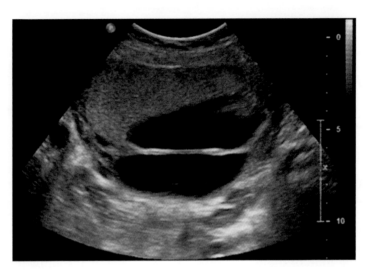

Figure 35.1 *Amniotic band.*

36

ABNORMALLY INVASIVE PLACENTA

An abnormally invasive placenta (AIP) is one of the most serious complications of pregnancy being associated with massive post-partum bleeding, high maternal morbidity and mortality, and a high frequency of post-partum hysterectomies. The condition is also sometimes termed as morbidly adherent placenta. Planned delivery at the right time, by the right multidisciplinary team, in the right place has the potential to improve maternal and fetal outcomes, and this can only be possible when AIP is suspected in the ante-natal period.

Risk factors

Risk factors can increase the likelihood of AIP but are not required for the diagnosis. These include advanced maternal age, assisted conception, and smoking. The associations of these risk factors are weak and do not form a good basis for a screening test.

Requirements

AIP is directly linked to previous Caesarean sections—in particular elective procedures where the scar is likely to be placed in the lower uterine segment rather than the cervical canal as with most emergency Caesarean sections in labor. The second requirement is a scar or uterine niche implantation (early pregnancy) which progresses to form a placenta praevia in the third trimester.

Ultrasound markers

Any woman with a previous Caesarean section (or uterine surgery) and a placenta praevia in this pregnancy should be assessed for an AIP in the early third trimester. The most reliable ultrasonographic markers of AIP are increased placental thickness and placental lacunae. Features such as loss of the normal hypoechoic retroplacental zone between the placenta and the uterus, bulging of the placenta into the posterior wall of the bladder, and increased color Doppler signals are less reproducible/reliable.

Bibliography

D'Antonio F, Iacovella C, Bhide A. Prenatal identification of invasive placentation using ultrasound: Systematic review and meta-analysis. *Ultrasound Obstet Gynecol* 2013; 42: 509–17.

Jauniaux E, Bhide A. Prenatal ultrasound diagnosis and outcome of placenta previa accreta after cesarean delivery: A systematic review and meta-analysis. *Am J Obstet Gynecol* 2017; 217: 27–36.

Jauniaux E, Bhide A, Kennedy A, Woodward P, Hubinont C, Collins S, for the FIGO Placenta Accreta Diagnosis and Management Expert Consensus Panel. FIGO consensus guidelines on placenta accreta spectrum disorders: Prenatal diagnosis and screening. *Int J Gynecol Obstet* 2018; 140:274–80.

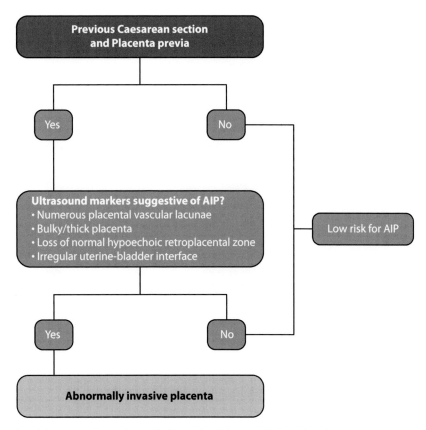

Algorithm 36.1 *Screening and diagnosis of abnormally invasive placenta.*

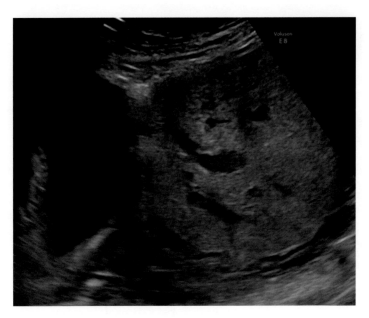

Figure 36.1 *Abnormally invasive placenta.*

37

HYDROPS

Fetal hydrops is defined as an abnormal accumulation of serous fluid in at least two fetal compartments—such as ascites, pleural or pericardial effusions, and skin edema. It is a non-specific finding due to a number of underlying abnormalities and is caused by an imbalance of fluid production and lymphatic return. This can be due to cardiac failure, obstructed lymphatic flow, or decreased plasma osmotic pressure. It is a rare condition, occurring in about 1 per 2000 births.

Hydrops can be divided into immune hydrops, which is due to hemolytic disease in the fetus secondary to maternal anti-red-cell atypical antibodies, and non-immune, which is due to all other causes. Although classically immune hydrops, and in particular rhesus disease, was the most common cause, the introduction of immunoglobulin prophylaxis in at-risk mothers has meant that non-immune causes have become relatively more common.

Hydrops is non-specific and can be due to a large number of underlying disorders, such as:

- Fetal anemia—alloimmune, parvovirus, hemorrhage, and hereditary anemias
- Fetal structural defects—cardiac defects, arrhythmias, and A-V malformations
- Thoracic compression—CCAM, sequestration, upper airway obstruction
- Fetal chromosomal abnormality or genetic syndromes
- Fetal metabolic disorder—glycogen and lysosome storage diseases
- Fetal congenital infection—cytomegalovirus, toxoplasmosis, and coxsackievirus

Management

This depends on the underlying cause. Fetal anemia due to immune causes can be treated by fetal blood transfusions to the fetus, with excellent survival rates and long-term outcome with appropriate treatment. Fetal anemia due to parvovirus infection or fetal-maternal hemorrhage can also often be treated by fetal blood transfusions. Fetal cardiac arrhythmias may be reversed by antiarrhythmic drugs, with resolution of hydrops in many cases. Hydrops due to compression by pleural effusions has been reported to have improved after pleuro-amniotic shunting.

Bibliography

Gajjar K, Spencer C. Diagnosis and management of non-anti-D red cell antibodies in pregnancy. *Obstet Gynaecol.* 2009; 11: 89–95.
Santo S, Mansour S, Thilaganathan B et al. Prenatal diagnosis of non-immune hydrops fetalis: What do we tell the parents? *Prenat Diagn.* 2011 Feb; 31(2): 186–95.

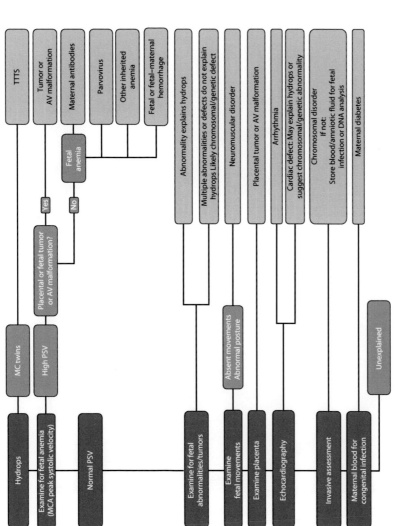

Algorithm 37.1 *Classification of hydrops. AV, arterio-venous; MC, monochorionic; MCA, middle cerebral artery; PSV, peak systolic velocity; TTTS, twin–twin transfusion syndrome.*

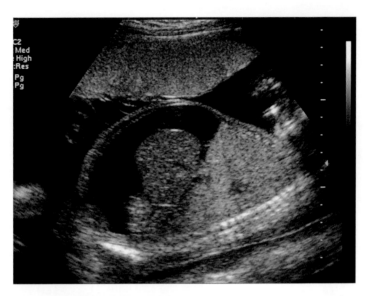

Figure 37.1 *Severe fetal hydrops.*

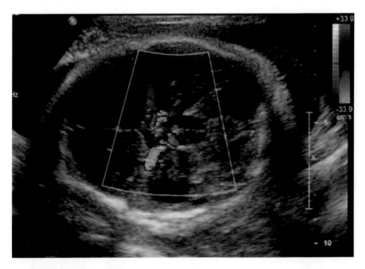

Figure 37.2 *Middle cerebral artery color Doppler.*

38

SMALL FETUS

A small-for-gestational-age (SGA) fetus is most commonly defined as a fetal size lower than the 10th percentile for gestational age. This group of babies is generally made up of fetuses that are normal (or constitutionally) small babies or those where the baby does not meet its growth potential—it has fetal growth restriction (FGR).

Diagnosis

SGA

Fetal measurements, usually of the abdominal circumference, are lower than the 10th percentile for gestational age.

FGR

FGR has been defined using an international consensus procedure and includes measures of size and fetal blood flow:

FGR (Early Onset)

The diagnosis is based on one of three solitary parameters (abdominal circumference [AC] <3rd centile, or estimated fetal weight [EFW] <3rd centile or absent end-diastolic flow in the umbilical artery [UA]) OR AC or EFW <10th centile combined with a pulsatility index (PI) >95th centile in either the umbilical or uterine artery.

FGR (Late Onset)

Abdominal circumference lower than the 3rd percentile, OR estimated fetal weight lower than the 3rd percentile, OR at least two out of three of the following:

- Abdominal circumference lower than the 10th percentile, OR estimated fetal weight lower than the 10th percentile
- Abdominal circumference OR estimated fetal weight crossing percentiles >2 quartiles
- Cerebro-placental ratio lower than the 5th percentile, OR pulsatility index in the umbilical artery higher than the 95th percentile

Causes

Broadly speaking, there are four reasons why fetal size may be small:

- Wrong gestational age
- A constitutionally or normal small fetus
- Poor placental function
- Some fetal abnormality

Wrong Dates

- Date the pregnancy from a previous good quality scan. Earlier scans will be more reliable, in particular if a fetal crown-rump length measurement was done between 9 and 14 weeks. *Once you have dated the pregnancy from this reliable, early scan, do not change the gestational age at later scans—this risks missing important growth abnormalities.*
- In cases where pregnancies are dated late or there is a question regarding the gestation, a scan in 3–4 weeks should be performed to ensure fetal growth continues on the same percentile. If there is a further fall in growth, consider an alternative diagnosis.

Constitutionally Small

- Normal uterine artery Dopplers, amniotic fluid, and Dopplers indices

Placental Insufficiency

- FGR is asymmetrical.
  - Usually, abdominal circumference more affected than femur length, followed by head circumference.
  - In cases of severe early onset growth restriction, the femur length may be the first to be affected.
- Doppler studies are abnormal, with the usual sequence of abnormal Doppler waveforms present first in the uterine, then the umbilical, and then the middle cerebral arteries. This is then followed by abnormal fetal venous Dopplers in the ductus venosus and finally umbilical veins, with antepartum fetal heart rate monitoring demonstrating reduced short-term variability (STV).
  - Uterine artery: High resistance to flow (high PI or RI, bilateral notches)
  - Umbilical artery: High resistance to flow (high PI or RI), may exhibit absent or reversed end-diastolic velocity
  - Middle cerebral artery: Low resistance to flow (low PI or RI), due to brain-sparing
  - Ductus venosus: High resistance to flow (high PIV), may exhibit absent or reversed a-wave

Fetal Abnormality

- The presence of FGR in the presence of fetal structural abnormalities, markers for chromosomal defects, or polyhydramnios makes the presence of congenital or acquired fetal abnormality likely.
- Causes include:
    - Chromosomal abnormality, most often triploidy, trisomy 18 or 13
    - Congenital fetal infections, e.g., Rubella, CMV, Toxoplasmosis
    - Fetal alcohol syndrome
    - Rarely genetic abnormality, e.g., uniparental disomy, Silver–Russell syndrome

Bibliography

Crino JP, Driggers RW. Ultrasound Findings Associated with Antepartum Viral Infection. *Clin Obstet Gynecol.* 2018 Mar; 61(1): 106–21.

Papageorghiou AT et al. International standards for fetal growth based on serial ultrasound measurements: the Fetal Growth Longitudinal Study of the INTERGROWTH-21st Project. *Lancet.* 2014 Sep 6; 384(9946): 869–879.

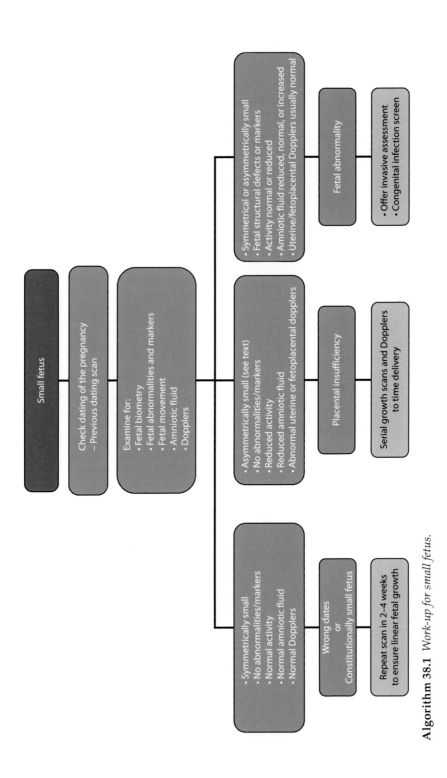

Algorithm 38.1 *Work-up for small fetus.*

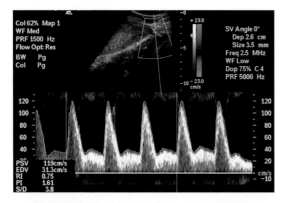

Figure 38.1 *High-resistance uterine artery Doppler.*

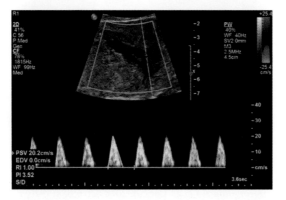

Figure 38.2 *Absent end-diastolic flow in the umbilical artery.*

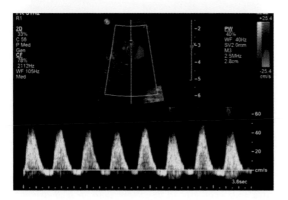

Figure 38.3 *Reversed end-diastolic flow in the umbilical artery.*

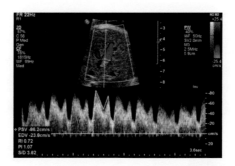

Figure 38.4 *High-resistance ductus venosus Doppler.*

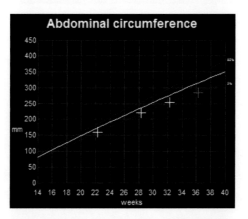

Figure 38.5 *Small fetus, but with normal fetal growth velocity.*
(From Papageorghiou AT et al. Lancet. *2014 Sep 6;384(9946):869–879.)*

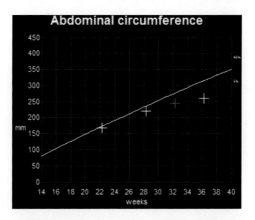

Figure 38.6 *Fetal growth restriction, with the fetal abdominal*
circumference gradually falling away from the expected normal range.
(From Papageorghiou AT et al. Lancet. *2014 Sep 6;384(9946):869–879.)*

39
TWIN-TO-TWIN TRANSFUSION SYNDROME

Approximately 22% of twin pregnancies are monochorionic (MC) and about 10%–15% of MC twin pregnancies are complicated by severe twin-to-twin transfusion syndrome (TTTS) as a result of a chronic circulatory imbalance in the vascular anastomoses that connect the fetuses. Chronic TTTS typically presents in the mid-second trimester with a host of maternal and perinatal findings. Chronic TTTS is progressive and is associated with a high rate of fetal loss if left untreated. Acute TTTS usually occurs in the third trimester and presents as polyhydramnios/oligohydramnios sequence. This is usually non-progressive and typically does not require intervention.

Prediction of TTTS

Although increased nuchal translucency has been reported as a marker for the subsequent development of TTTS, this has not been borne out in larger series. However, folding of the intertwin membrane can be identified at 15–17 weeks of gestation as an early manifestation of disparity in amniotic fluid volume and is associated with the development of severe TTTS in about 25% of cases.

Diagnosis of TTTS

Chronic TTTS is diagnosed prenatally on the identification of the donor twin presenting with oligohydramnios or anhydramnios and the recipient twin simultaneously having polyhydramnios. The donor appears to be stuck with a lower estimated fetal weight and an absent or small fetal bladder. The recipient appears to be of either average or above average weight with a big bladder. Doppler changes may accompany these findings and usually signify worsening TTTS. The donor twin may have absent or reversed end-diastolic flow in the umbilical artery Doppler. Additional features include hypertrophic heart with poor contractility in the recipient. With worsening TTTS, the recipient may present with hydrops.

Staging of TTTS

Attempts have been made to stage the process in TTTS; however, the relationship of this staging to the natural history and outcome of TTTS remains to be established.

Management of TTTS

Laser photocoagulation involves the introduction of a laser fiber through a fetoscope into the recipient's sac under ultrasound guidance. The intertwin anastomoses are photocoagulated on the placental surface and the excess amniotic fluid is drained at the end of the procedure. Fetoscopic laser coagulation of the anastomoses currently results in 66%–82% survival rate in at least one twin. Adverse neurological sequelae have been reported in approximately 5% of survivors.

Bibliography

Khalil A, Rodgers M, Baschat A et al. ISUOG Practice Guidelines: Role of ultrasound in twin pregnancy. *Ultrasound Obstet Gynecol*. 2016 Feb; 47(2): 247–63.

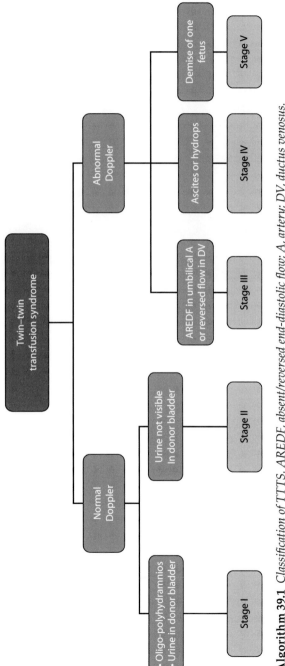

Algorithm 39.1 *Classification of TTTS. AREDF, absent/reversed end-diastolic flow; A, artery; DV, ductus venosus.*

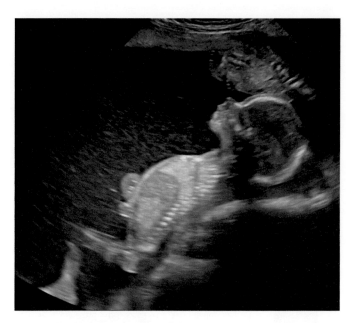

Figure 39.1 *TTTS: recipient twin with polyhydramnios, donor twin stuck with no fluid.*

INDEX